QUICK · EASY
HEALTHY

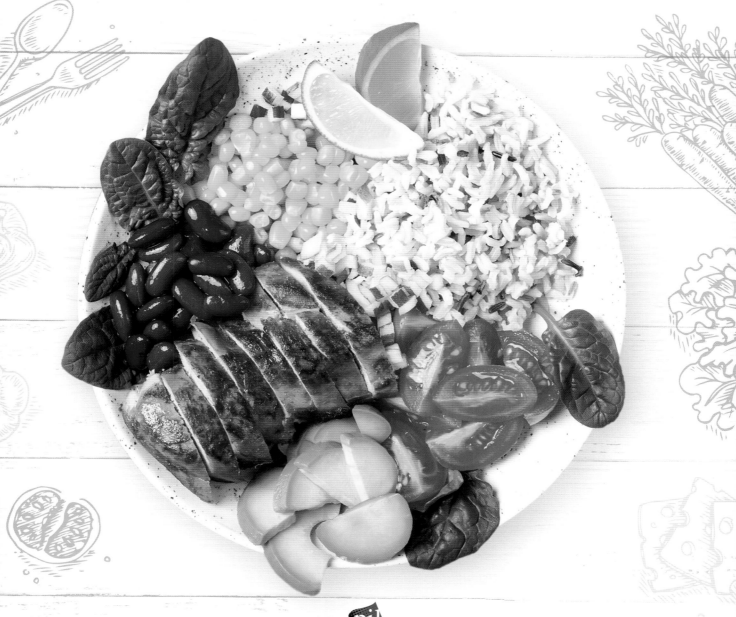

Publications International, Ltd.

Photo on front cover © Shutterstock.com

Artwork on cover, endsheets, and pages 5, 29, 53, 71, 139, and 167 © Shutterstock.com

Pictured on the front cover: Fajita-Seasoned Grilled Chicken Bowl (*page 74*).

Pictured on the back cover (*from top to bottom*): Carrot Raisin Salad with Citrus Dressing (*page 158*) and Fruit Salad with Creamy Banana Dressing (*page 188*).

ISBN: 978-1-64030-448-2

Manufactured in China.

8   7   6   5   4   3   2   1

Microwave Cooking: Microwave ovens vary in wattage. Use the cooking times as guidelines and check for doneness before adding more time.

Nutritional Analysis: Every effort has been made to check the accuracy of the nutritional information that appears with each recipe. However, because numerous variables account for a wide range of values for certain foods, nutritive analyses in this book should be considered approximate.

WARNING: Food preparation, baking and cooking involve inherent dangers: misuse of electric products, sharp electric tools, boiling water, hot stoves, allergic reactions, foodborne illnesses and the like, pose numerous potential risks. Publications International, Ltd. (PIL) assumes no responsibility or liability for any damages you may experience as a result of following recipes, instructions, tips or advice in this publication.

While we hope this publication helps you find new ways to eat delicious foods, you may not always achieve the results desired due to variations in ingredients, cooking temperatures, typos, errors, omissions, or individual cooking abilities.

TABLE OF CONTENTS

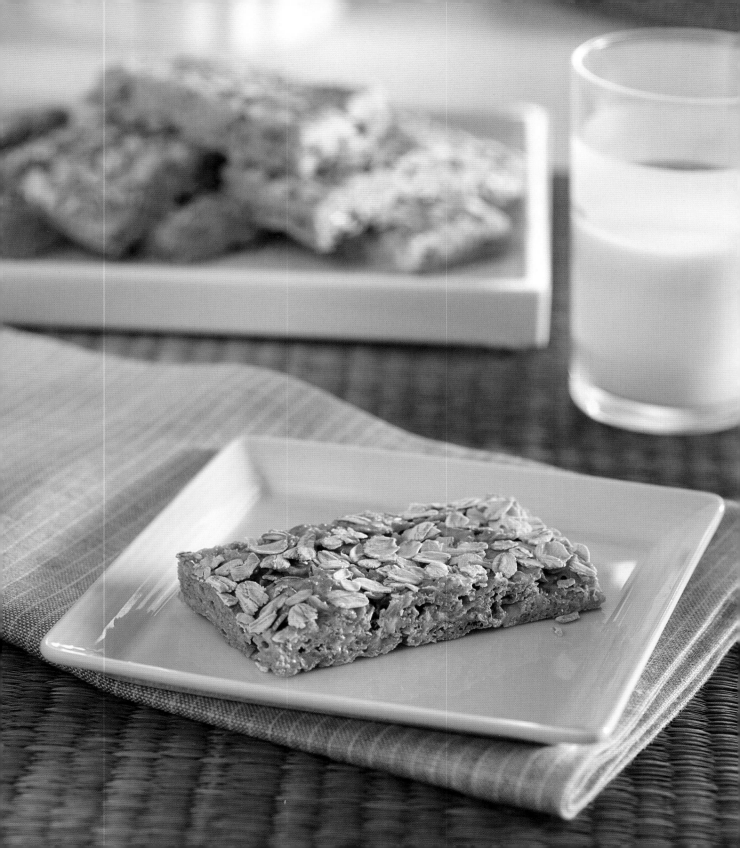

APPETIZERS & SNACKS

WHOLE-GRAIN CEREAL BARS

Makes 24 bars

5 to 6 cups assorted whole grain cereals

1 package (10 ounces) large marshmallows

¼ cup (½ stick) butter

¼ cup old-fashioned oats

1. Grease 13×19-inch baking pan.

2. Place cereals in large resealable food storage bag; seal bag. Using rolling pin, lightly roll over bag until cereals are crumbled.

3. Combine marshmallows and butter in large saucepan over medium-low heat; cook and stir until marshmallows are melted and mixture is smooth. Remove from heat.

4. Stir in cereal until well blended. Using waxed paper, press cereal mixture evenly into prepared pan. Sprinkle with oats. Let stand until firm. Cut into bars.

NUTRITIONAL INFORMATION

Calories **88**, Total Fat **2g**, Saturated Fat **1g**, Cholesterol **5mg**, Sodium **76mg**, Carbohydrates **17g**, Dietary Fiber **1g**, Protein **1g**

EASY NACHOS

Makes 4 servings

4 (6-inch) flour tortillas

Nonstick cooking spray

¼ pound 93% lean ground turkey

⅔ cup salsa

2 tablespoons sliced green onion

½ cup (2 ounces) shredded reduced-fat Cheddar cheese

1. Preheat oven to 350°F. Cut each tortilla into 8 wedges; lightly spray one side of wedges with cooking spray. Place on ungreased baking sheet. Bake 5 to 9 minutes or until lightly browned and crisp.

2. Meanwhile, brown turkey in small nonstick skillet over medium-high heat, stirring to break up meat; drain fat. Stir in salsa; cook until heated through.

3. Spoon turkey mixture evenly over tortilla wedges. Sprinkle with green onion. Top with cheese. Bake 1 to 2 minutes or until cheese melts.

SERVING SUGGESTION: To make these nachos even more special, cut tortillas into shapes with cookie cutters and bake as directed.

TIP: In a hurry? Substitute baked corn chips for flour tortillas and cooking spray. Proceed as directed.

NUTRITIONAL INFORMATION

Calories **190**, Total Fat **7g**, Saturated Fat **3g**, Cholesterol **25mg**, Sodium **580mg**, Carbohydrates **20g**, Dietary Fiber **2g**, Protein **13g**

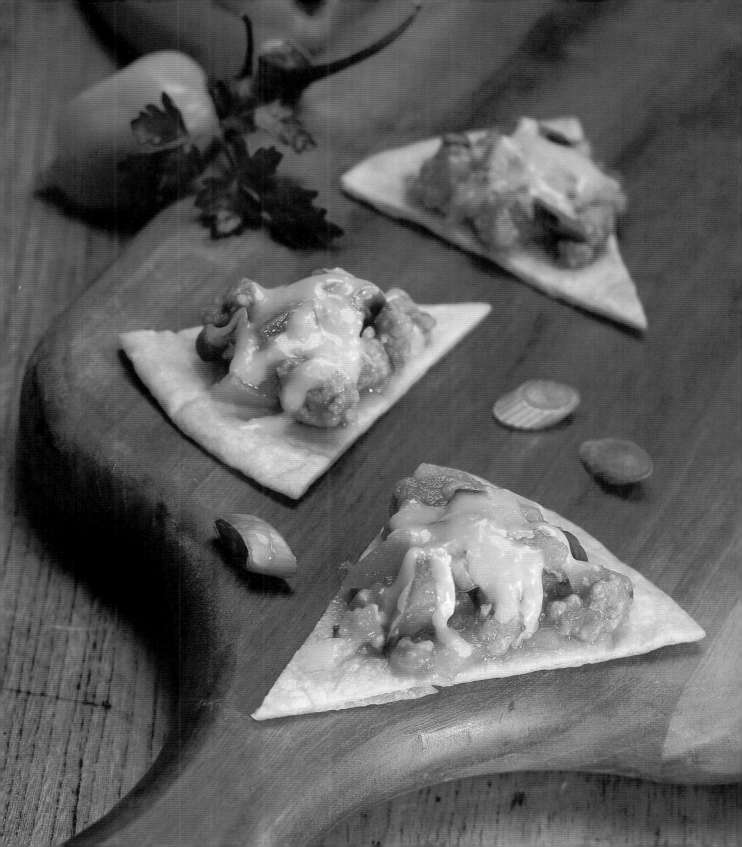

GREAT ZUKES PIZZA BITES

Makes 8 servings (2 bites per serving)

1 medium zucchini

3 tablespoons pizza sauce

2 tablespoons tomato paste

¼ teaspoon dried oregano

¾ cup (3 ounces) shredded mozzarella cheese

¼ cup shredded Parmesan cheese

8 slices pitted black olives

8 slices pepperoni

1. Preheat broiler; set rack 4 inches from heat.

2. Trim off and discard ends of zucchini. Cut zucchini into 16 (¼-inch-thick) diagonal slices. Place on nonstick baking sheet.

3. Combine pizza sauce, tomato paste and oregano in small bowl; mix well. Spread scant teaspoon sauce over each zucchini slice. Combine cheeses in small bowl. Top each zucchini slice with 1 tablespoon cheese mixture, pressing down into sauce. Place 1 olive slice on each of 8 pizza bites. Place 1 folded pepperoni slice on each remaining pizza bite.

4. Broil 3 minutes or until cheese is melted. Serve immediately.

NUTRITIONAL INFORMATION

Calories **75**, Total Fat **5g**, Saturated Fat **2g**, Cholesterol **10mg**, Sodium **288mg**, Carbohydrates **3g**, Dietary Fiber **1g**, Protein **5g**

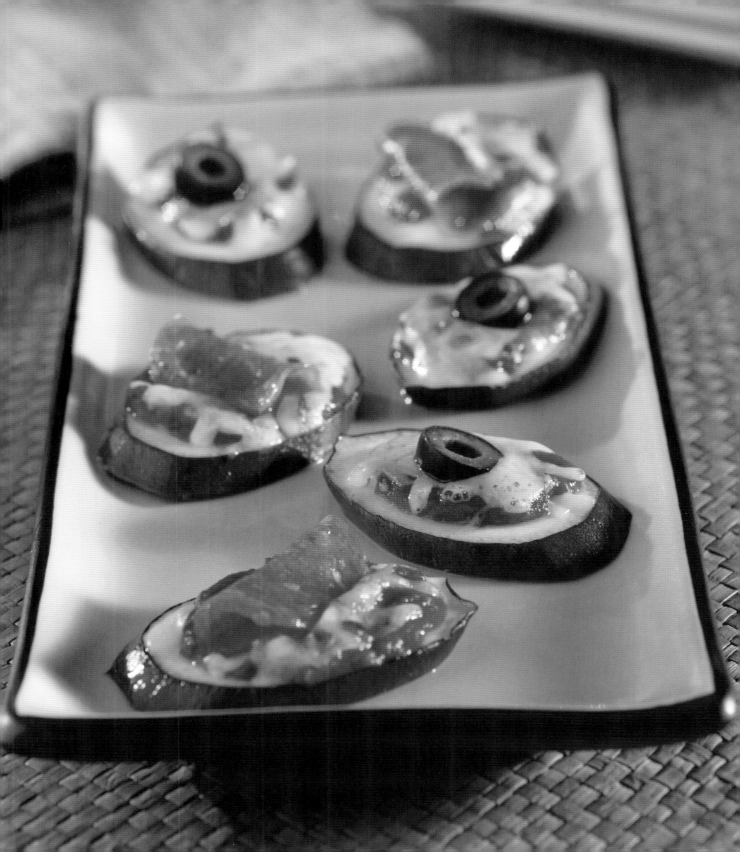

FRUIT KABOBS WITH RASPBERRY YOGURT DIP

Makes 6 servings

½ cup plain nonfat yogurt

¼ cup no-sugar-added raspberry fruit spread

1 pint fresh strawberries

2 cups cubed honeydew melon (1-inch cubes)

2 cups cubed cantaloupe (1-inch cubes)

1 can (8 ounces) pineapple chunks in juice, drained

1. Stir yogurt and fruit spread in small bowl until well blended.

2. Thread fruit alternately onto six 12-inch skewers. Serve with yogurt dip.

NUTRITIONAL INFORMATION

Calories **108**, Total Fat **1g**, Saturated Fat **1g**, Cholesterol **1mg**, Sodium **52mg**, Carbohydrates **25g**, Dietary Fiber **2g**, Protein **2g**

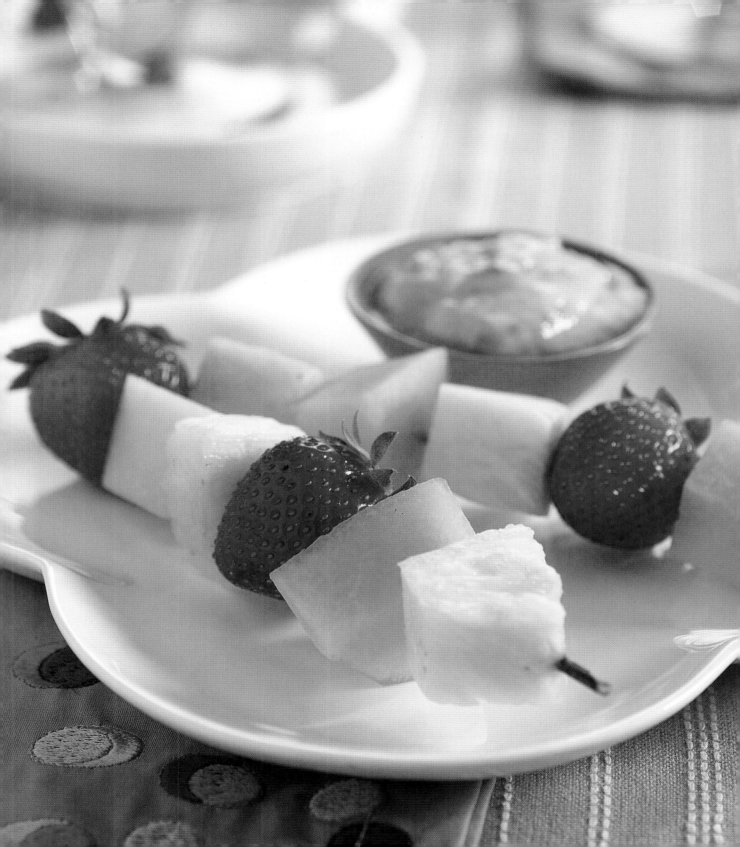

ASIAN VEGETABLE ROLLS WITH SOY-LIME DIPPING SAUCE

Makes 6 servings (3 rolls per serving)

¼ cup reduced-sodium soy sauce

2 tablespoons lime juice

1 clove garlic, crushed

1 teaspoon honey

½ teaspoon finely chopped fresh ginger

¼ teaspoon dark sesame oil

⅛ to ¼ teaspoon red pepper flakes

½ cup grated cucumber

⅓ cup grated carrot

¼ cup sliced yellow bell pepper (1 inch long)

2 tablespoons thinly sliced green onion

18 small lettuce leaves

Sesame seeds (optional)

1. Combine soy sauce, lime juice, garlic, honey, ginger, oil and red pepper flakes in small bowl.

2. Combine cucumber, carrot, bell pepper and green onion in medium bowl. Stir in 1 tablespoon soy sauce mixture.

3. Place about 1 tablespoon vegetable mixture on each lettuce leaf. Roll up leaves; sprinkle with sesame seeds, if desired. Serve with remaining sauce for dipping.

NUTRITIONAL INFORMATION

Calories **25**, Total Fat **1g**, Saturated Fat **1g**, Cholesterol **0mg**, Sodium **343mg**, Carbohydrates **5g**, Dietary Fiber **1g**, Protein **1g**

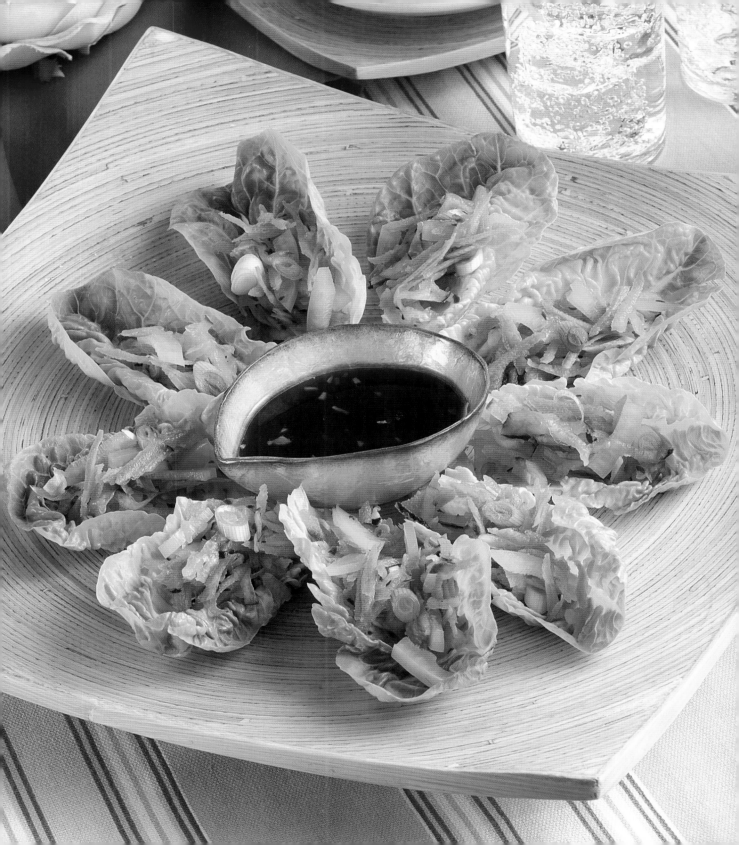

CINNAMON TRAIL MIX

Makes 8 (¾-cup) servings

2 cups corn cereal squares

2 cups whole wheat cereal squares or whole wheat cereal squares with mini graham crackers

1½ cups fat-free oyster crackers

½ cup broken sesame snack sticks

2 tablespoons butter, melted

1 teaspoon ground cinnamon

¼ teaspoon ground nutmeg

½ cup fruit-flavored candy pieces

1. Preheat oven to 350°F. Spray 13×9-inch baking pan with nonstick cooking spray.

2. Place cereals, crackers and sesame sticks in prepared pan; mix lightly.

3. Combine butter, cinnamon and nutmeg in small bowl; mix well. Drizzle evenly over cereal mixture; toss to coat.

4. Bake 12 to 14 minutes or until golden brown, stirring gently after 6 minutes. Cool completely. Stir in candies.

NUTRITIONAL INFORMATION

Calories **280**, Total Fat **8g**, Saturated Fat **1g**, Cholesterol **0mg**, Sodium **515mg**, Carbohydrates **47g**, Dietary Fiber **3g**, Protein **5g**

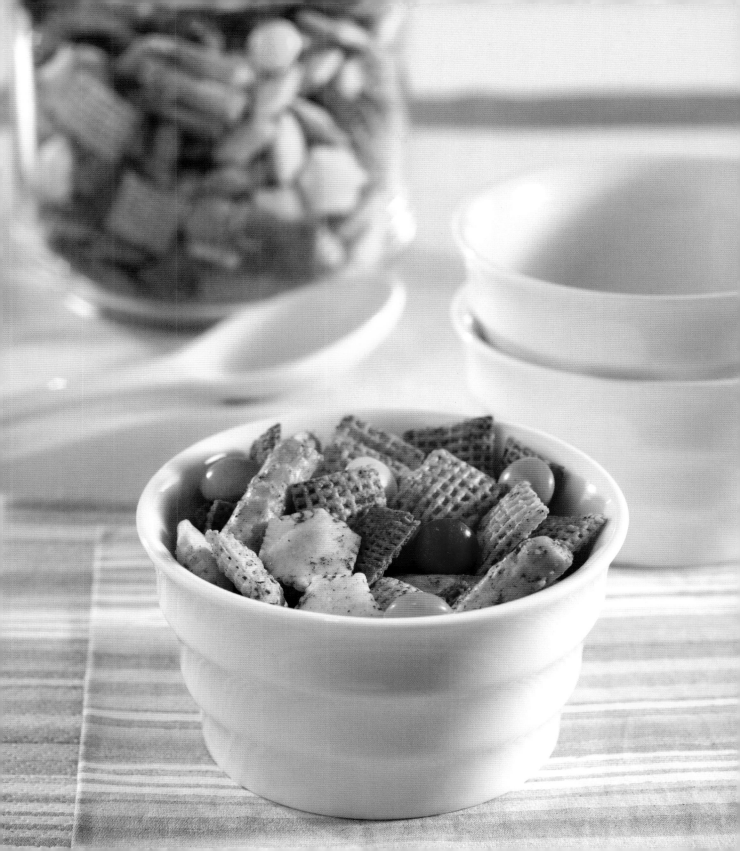

SARA'S GUILTLESS ARTICHOKE DIP

Makes 2 cups (about 16 servings)

8 light garlic-and-herb spreadable cheese wedges

1 can (about 14 ounces) artichokes packed in water, rinsed, drained and coarsely chopped

½ cup (2 ounces) shredded reduced-fat mozzarella cheese

¼ cup shredded Parmesan cheese

1 tablespoon light sour cream, plus additional if necessary

2 teaspoons fresh lemon juice

¼ teaspoon ground red pepper

Assorted vegetable sticks, pretzel chips and/or crackers

MICROWAVE DIRECTIONS

1. Stir cheese wedges in medium microwavable bowl until smooth. Add artichokes, mozzarella cheese, Parmesan cheese, 1 tablespoon sour cream, lemon juice and red pepper. Add additional sour cream, if necessary, to thin dip to desired consistency.

2. Microwave on HIGH 1 minute; stir. Microwave at 30-second intervals until heated through, stirring after each interval.

3. Serve with assorted vegetable sticks, pretzel chips and/or crackers.

NUTRITIONAL INFORMATION

Calories **46**, Total Fat **2g**, Saturated Fat **1g**, Cholesterol **4mg**, Sodium **215mg**, Carbohydrates **3g**, Dietary Fiber **1g**, Protein **3g**

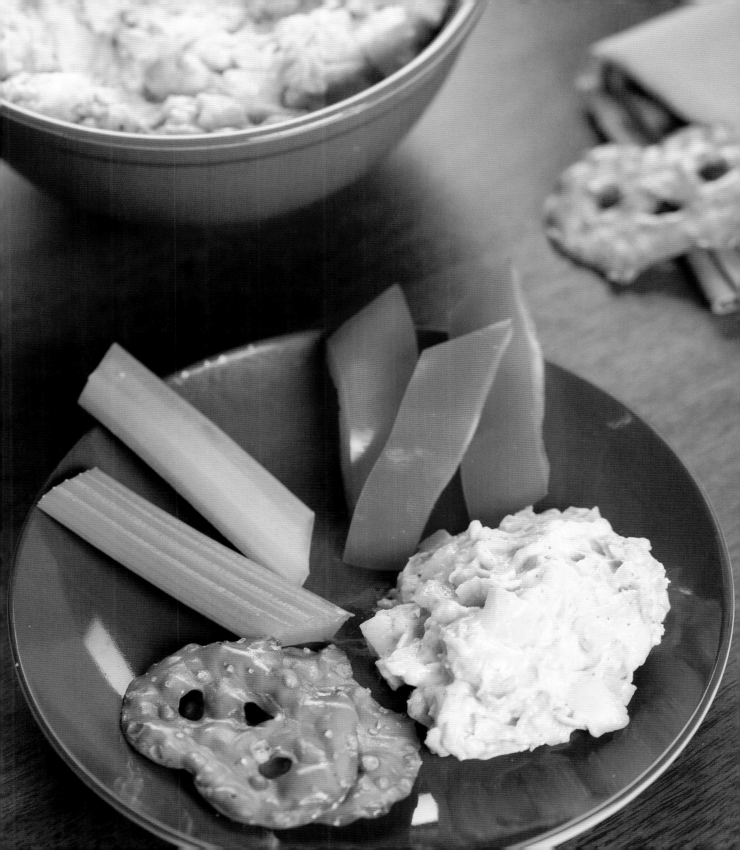

SNACK ATTACK MIX

Makes 16 (½ cup) servings

4 cups unsweetened corn cereal squares or whole wheat cereal squares

1½ ounces (¾ cup) fat-free pretzels sticks, broken in half

1½ ounces (1 cup) multigrain pita chips, broken into bite-size pieces

4 ounces (about 1 cup) slivered almonds

2 teaspoons paprika

1 teaspoon dry mustard

1 teaspoon garlic powder

1 teaspoon salt

½ teaspoon ground cumin

¼ teaspoon ground red pepper

2 tablespoons Worcestershire sauce

2 teaspoons canola oil

1½ teaspoons cider vinegar

1. Preheat oven to 300°F. Combine cereal, pretzels, pita chips and almonds in large bowl; set aside.

2. Combine remaining ingredients in small bowl; stir until well blended. Spoon over cereal mixture; toss gently, yet thoroughly to coat completely. Spread evenly on large baking sheet. Bake 10 to 15 minutes or until beginning to lightly brown, stirring every 5 minutes.

3. Remove from oven; place baking sheet on wire rack. Let stand 2 hours. Store leftovers in an airtight container at room temperature.

NUTRITIONAL INFORMATION

Calories **99**, Total Fat **5g**, Saturated Fat **0g**, Cholesterol **0mg**, Sodium **279mg**, Carbohydrates **12g**, Dietary Fiber **2g**, Protein **3g**

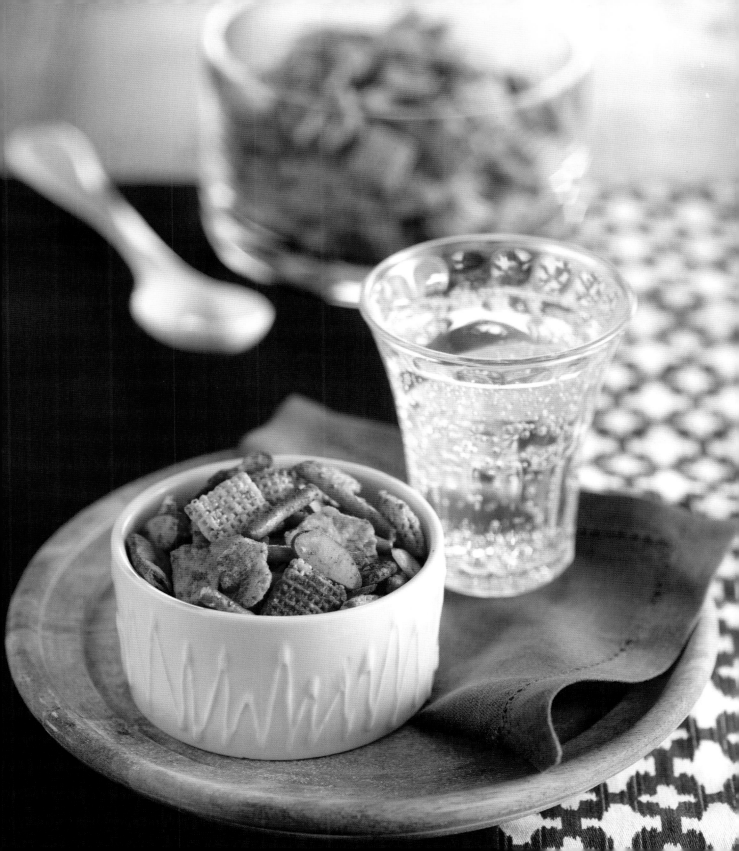

MEDITERRANEAN TUNA CUPS

Makes 10 servings (3 cups per serving)

3 English cucumbers

⅔ cup plain nonfat Greek yogurt

⅓ cup coarsely chopped pitted kalamata olives

⅓ cup finely chopped red onion

2 tablespoons fresh lemon juice

¼ teaspoon garlic salt

2 cans (5 ounces each) solid white albacore tuna in water, drained and flaked

1. Cut ends off of each cucumber; cut each cucumber into 10 slices. Scoop out cucumber slices with rounded ½ teaspoon, leaving thick shell.

2. Stir yogurt, olives, onion, lemon juice and garlic salt in large bowl until smooth and well blended. Stir in tuna.

3. Spoon about 1 tablespoon tuna salad into each cucumber cup. Serve immediately.

NUTRITIONAL INFORMATION

Calories **32**, Total Fat **1g**, Saturated Fat **0g**, Cholesterol **8mg**, Sodium **102mg**, Carbohydrates **2g**, Dietary Fiber **1g**, Protein **5g**

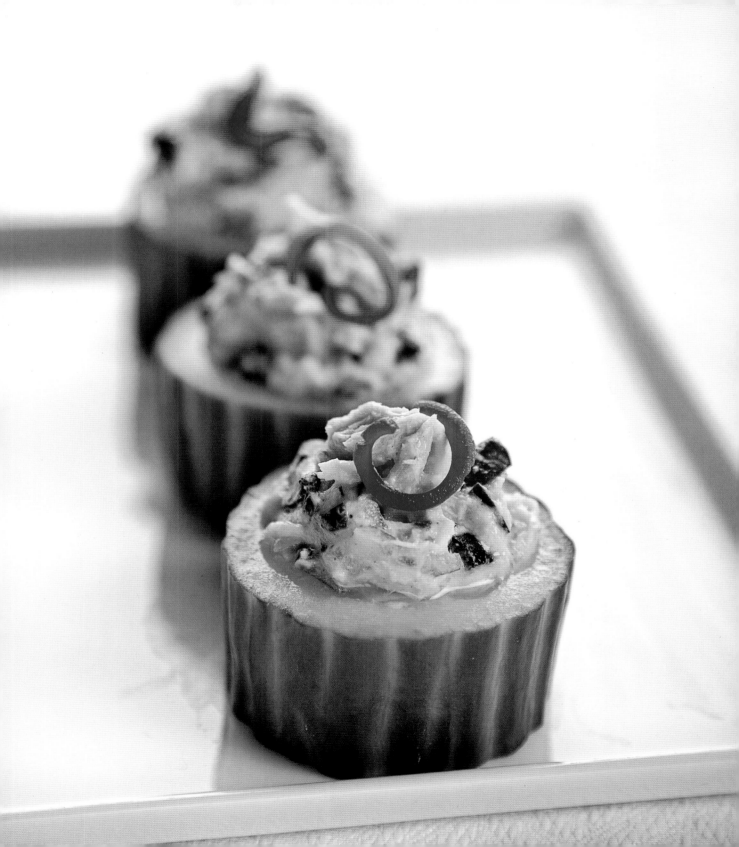

CHOCO-PEANUT BUTTER POPCORN

Makes 6 (⅔-cup) servings

⅓ cup semisweet chocolate chips

3 tablespoons natural creamy peanut butter

1 tablespoon butter spread

4 cups air-popped popcorn

½ cup powdered sugar

MICROWAVE DIRECTIONS

1. Microwave chocolate chips, peanut butter and butter in medium microwavable bowl on HIGH 30 seconds; stir. Microwave 30 seconds or until melted and smooth. Pour mixture over popcorn in large bowl, stirring until evenly coated. Transfer to 1-gallon resealable food storage bag.

2. Add powdered sugar to bag; seal bag. Shake until well coated. Spread onto waxed paper to cool. Store leftovers in airtight container in refrigerator.

NUTRITIONAL INFORMATION

Calories **161**, Total Fat **9g**, Saturated Fat **3g**, Cholesterol **5mg**, Sodium **19mg**, Carbohydrates **20g**, Dietary Fiber **2g**, Protein **3g**

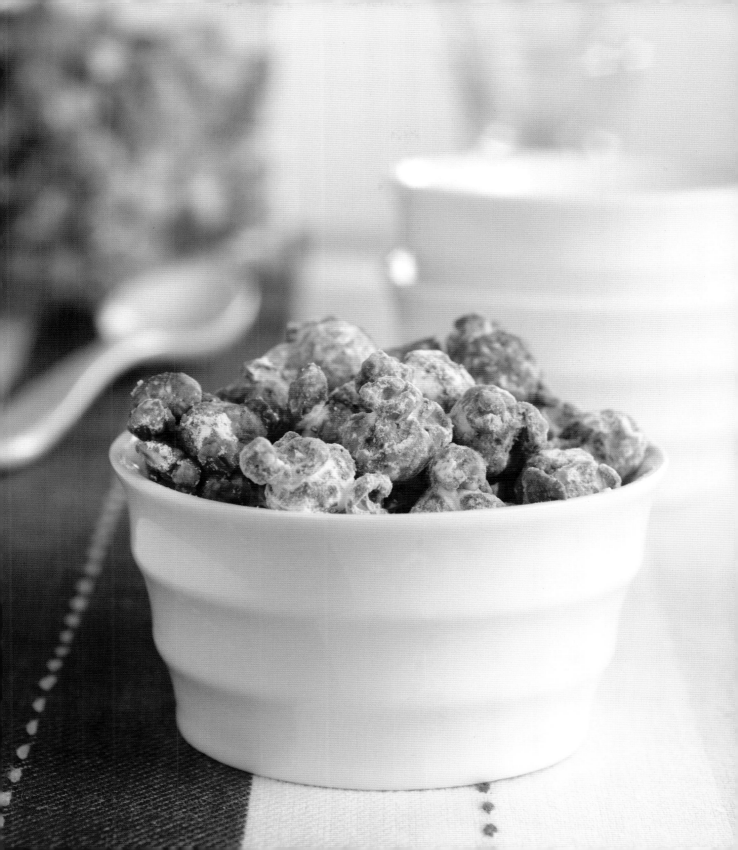

MINI CHEESE BURRITOS

Makes 4 servings

½ cup canned fat-free refried beans

4 (8-inch) flour tortillas

½ cup chunky salsa

4 (¾-ounce) reduced-fat Cheddar cheese sticks*

*Reduced-fat Cheddar cheese block can be substituted. Cut cheese into sticks.

MICROWAVE DIRECTIONS

1. Spread beans over tortillas, leaving ½ inch border around edges. Spoon salsa over beans.

2. Place cheese stick on one side of each tortilla. Fold edge of tortilla over cheese stick; roll up. Place burritos, seam side down, in microwavable dish.

3. Microwave on HIGH 1 to 2 minutes or until cheese is melted. Let stand 1 to 2 minutes before serving.

NUTRITIONAL INFORMATION

Calories **109**, Total Fat **4g**, Saturated Fat **3g**, Cholesterol **10mg**, Sodium **435mg**, Carbohydrates **11g**, Dietary Fiber **4g**, Protein **9g**

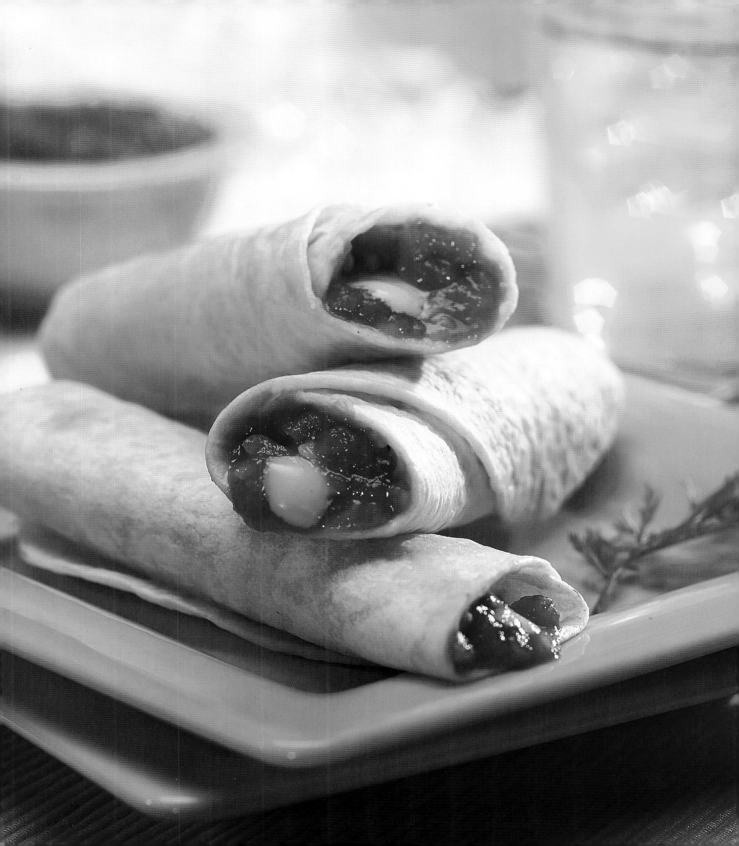

CROSTINI

Makes 8 servings (2 crostini per serving)

1 whole wheat mini baguette
(about 4 ounces)

4 plum tomatoes

1 cup (4 ounces) shredded
part-skim mozzarella cheese

3 tablespoons pesto sauce

1. Preheat oven to 400°F. Slice baguette into 16 very thin, diagonal slices. Slice each tomato lengthwise into 4 (¼-inch) slices.

2. Place baguette slices on ungreased baking sheet. Top each with 1 tablespoon cheese and 1 tomato slice.

3. Bake 8 minutes or until bread is lightly toasted and cheese is melted. Top each crostini with about ½ teaspoon pesto sauce. Serve warm.

NUTRITIONAL INFORMATION

Calories **83**, Total Fat **3g**, Saturated Fat **2g**, Cholesterol **9mg**, Sodium **159mg**, Carbohydrates **9g**, Dietary Fiber **1g**, Protein **5g**

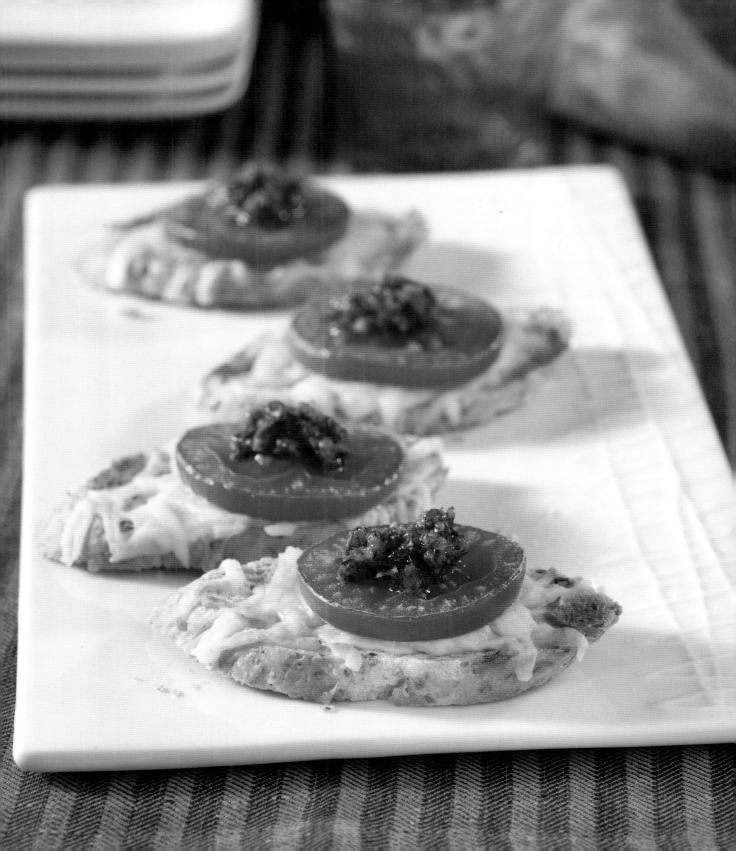

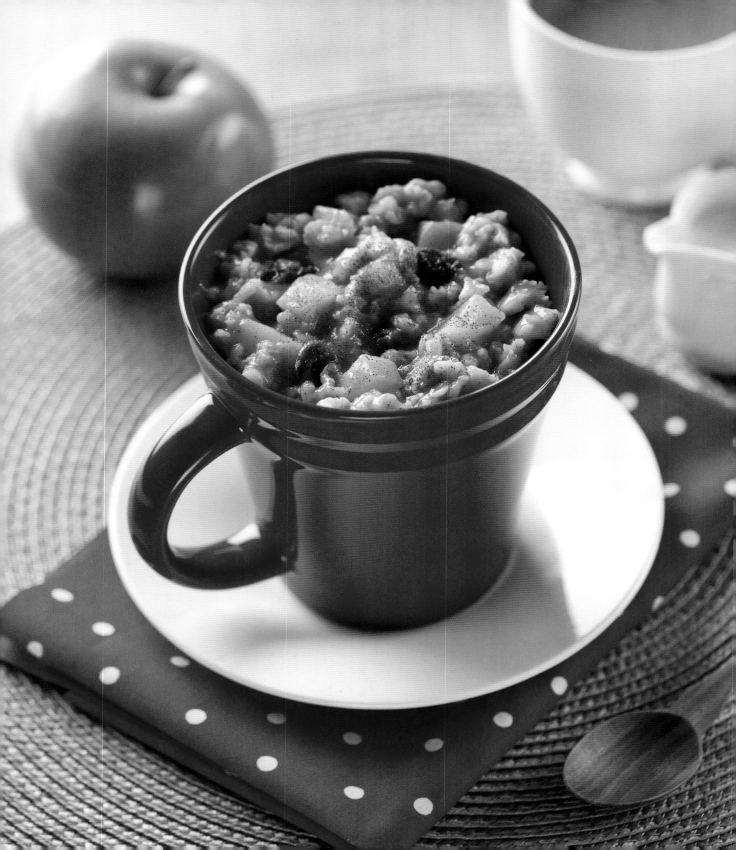

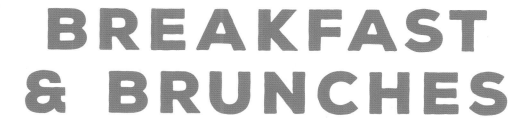

BREAKFAST & BRUNCHES

HARVEST APPLE OATMUG

Makes 1 serving

1 cup water

½ cup old-fashioned oats

½ cup chopped Granny Smith apple

2 tablespoons raisins

1 teaspoon packed brown sugar

¼ teaspoon ground cinnamon

⅛ teaspoon salt

MICROWAVE DIRECTIONS

1. Combine water, oats, apple, raisins, brown sugar, cinnamon and salt in large microwavable mug; mix well.

2. Microwave on HIGH 1½ minutes; stir. Microwave on HIGH 1 minute or until thickened and liquid is absorbed. Let stand 1 to 2 minutes before serving.

NUTRITIONAL INFORMATION

Calories **251**, Total Fat **3g**, Saturated Fat **1g**, Cholesterol **0mg**, Sodium **302mg**, Carbohydrates **54g**, Dietary Fiber **6g**, Protein **6g**

BREAKFAST PIZZA MARGHERITA

Makes 6 servings

1 (12-inch) prepared pizza crust

3 slices 95% fat-free turkey bacon

2 cups cholesterol-free egg substitute

½ cup fat-free (skim) milk

1½ tablespoons chopped fresh basil, divided

⅛ teaspoon black pepper

2 plum tomatoes, thinly sliced

½ cup (2 ounces) shredded reduced-fat mozzarella cheese

¼ cup (1 ounce) shredded reduced-fat Cheddar cheese

1. Preheat oven to 450°F. Place pizza crust on 12-inch pizza pan. Bake 6 to 8 minutes or until heated through.

2. Meanwhile, coat large skillet with nonstick cooking spray. Cook bacon over medium-high heat until crisp. Remove from skillet to paper towels; cool. Crumble bacon.

3. Combine egg substitute, milk, ½ tablespoon basil and pepper in medium bowl. Coat same skillet with cooking spray. Add egg substitute mixture. Cook over medium heat until mixture begins to set around edges. Gently stir eggs, allowing uncooked portions to flow underneath. Repeat stirring of egg mixture every 1 to 2 minutes or until eggs are just set. Remove from heat.

4. Arrange tomato slices on warmed pizza crust. Spoon scrambled eggs over tomatoes. Sprinkle with bacon. Top with cheeses. Bake 1 minute or until cheese is melted. Sprinkle with remaining 1 tablespoon basil. Cut into 6 wedges. Serve immediately.

NUTRITIONAL INFORMATION

Calories **311**, Total Fat **9g**, Saturated Fat **2g**, Cholesterol **11mg**, Sodium **675mg**, Carbohydrates **35g**, Dietary Fiber **2g**, Protein **21g**

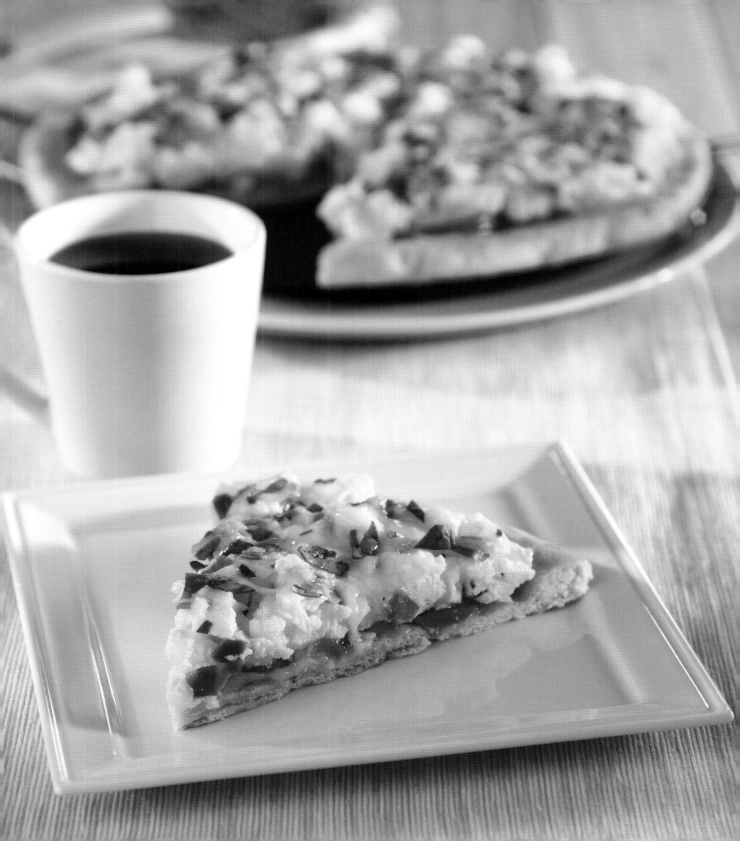

NUTMEG PANCAKES WITH LEMON-SPIKED BERRIES

Makes 6 servings

1 cup all-purpose flour

2 tablespoons sugar substitute,* divided

1 teaspoon baking powder

¾ teaspoon ground nutmeg

½ teaspoon baking soda

¼ teaspoon salt

1⅓ cups nonfat buttermilk

¼ cup cholesterol-free egg substitute

2 tablespoons canola oil

2 cups sliced strawberries

2 teaspoons grated lemon peel

This recipe was tested with sucralose-based sugar substitute.

1. Combine flour, 1 tablespoon sugar substitute, baking powder, nutmeg, baking soda and salt in medium bowl. Combine buttermilk, egg substitute and oil in small bowl. Add to flour mixture; stir just until moistened.

2. Lightly spray nonstick griddle with nonstick cooking spray; heat over medium-high heat. For each pancake, pour about ¼ cup batter onto hot griddle. Cook until top is covered with bubbles and edge is slightly dry. Turn pancake; cook until done.

3. Meanwhile, combine strawberries, remaining 1 tablespoon sugar substitute and lemon peel in medium bowl. Serve strawberry mixture over warm pancakes.

NUTRITIONAL INFORMATION

Calories **162**, Total Fat **5g**, Saturated Fat **1g**, Cholesterol **2mg**, Sodium **361mg**, Carbohydrates **23g**, Dietary Fiber **2g**, Protein **5g**

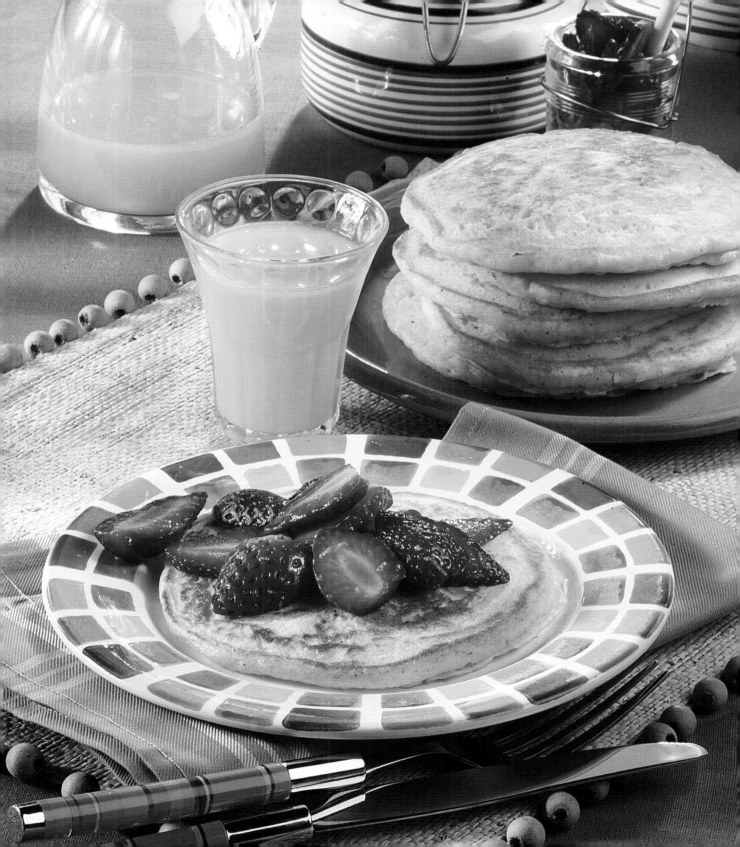

BUCKWHEAT BREAKFAST BOWL

Makes 6 servings

3 to 4 cups reduced-fat (2%) milk*

2 tablespoons packed brown sugar

½ teaspoon vanilla

½ teaspoon ground cinnamon, divided

1 cup kasha**

2 teaspoons butter

2 apples, thinly sliced

2 tablespoons maple syrup

¼ cup chopped walnuts

For a creamier consistency, use more milk.

**Kasha, or buckwheat groats, is buckwheat that has been pre-toasted. It is commonly found in the Kosher section of the supermarket.*

1. Combine milk, brown sugar, vanilla and ¼ teaspoon cinnamon in large saucepan. Bring to a boil over medium heat. Stir in kasha; reduce heat to low. Cook and stir 8 to 10 minutes or until kasha is tender and liquid is absorbed.

2. Meanwhile, melt butter in large nonstick skillet over medium heat. Stir in remaining ¼ teaspoon cinnamon. Add apples; cook and stir 4 to 5 minutes or until tender. Stir in maple syrup and walnuts; heat through.

3. Spoon kasha into six bowls. Top with apple mixture. Serve immediately.

NUTRITIONAL INFORMATION

Calories **226**, Total Fat **8g**, Saturated Fat **3g**, Cholesterol **13mg**, Sodium **119mg**, Carbohydrates **34g**, Dietary Fiber **3g**, Protein **6g**

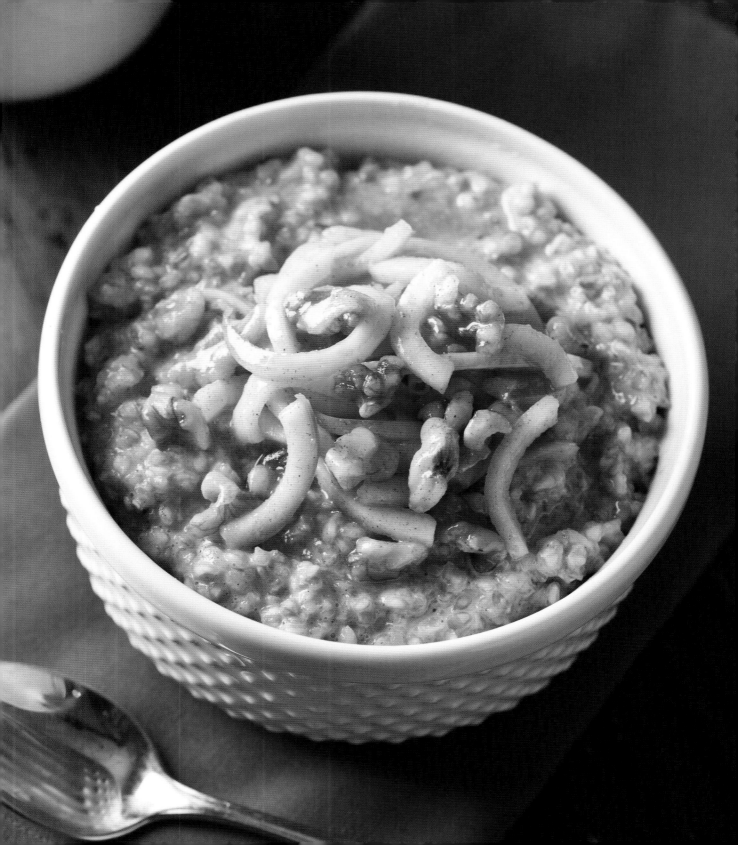

BREAKFAST QUESADILLAS

Makes 4 servings (2 quesadillas per serving)

1 cup cholesterol-free egg substitute

2 tablespoons fat-free (skim) milk

4 teaspoons canola oil, divided

1 can (4 ounces) chopped mild green chiles

8 soft corn tortillas

½ cup (2 ounces) shredded reduced-fat sharp Cheddar cheese

¼ cup chopped fresh cilantro

1 ounce turkey pepperoni slices, quartered

1. Whisk egg substitute and milk in small bowl. Heat 2 teaspoons oil in large skillet over medium heat. Cook eggs until set, lifting edges to allow uncooked portion to flow underneath. Remove from skillet. Wipe out skillet with paper towel.

2. Spread 1 tablespoon chiles on half of each tortilla. Top each with eggs, cheese and cilantro; sprinkle evenly with pepperoni. Fold tortillas in half.

3. Heat remaining 2 teaspoons oil in skillet. Cook quesadillas in two batches 3 minutes per side or until cheese is melted.

NUTRITIONAL INFORMATION

Calories **246**, Total Fat **10g**, Saturated Fat **3g**, Cholesterol **19mg**, Sodium **490mg**, Carbohydrates **25g**, Dietary Fiber **3g**, Protein **15g**

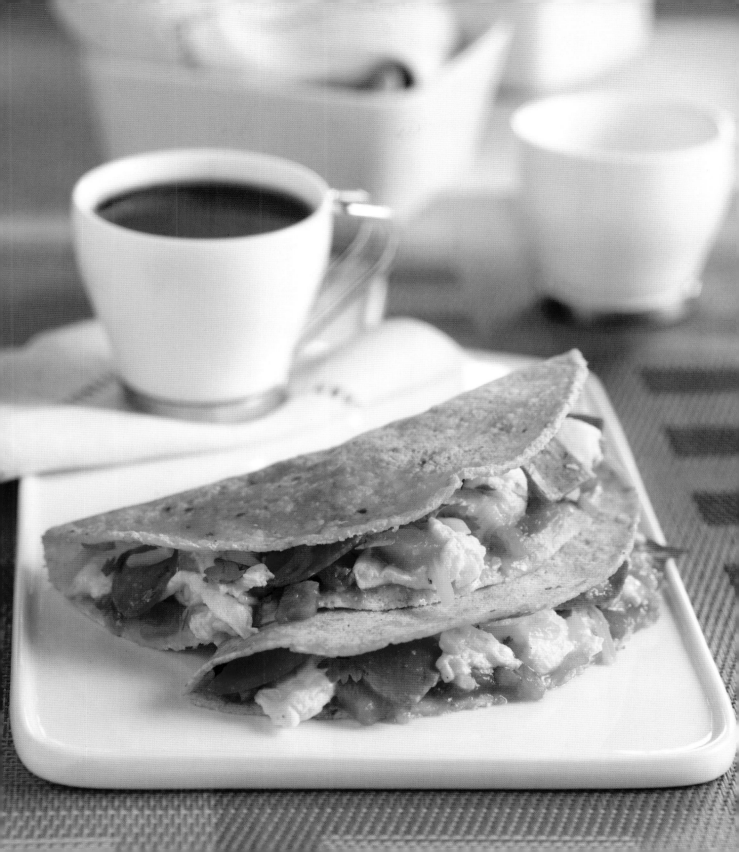

VERY BERRY YOGURT PARFAITS

Makes 4 servings

3 cups plain nonfat yogurt

2 tablespoons sugar-free berry preserves

1 packet sugar substitute*

½ teaspoon vanilla

2 cups sliced fresh strawberries

1 cup fresh blueberries

4 tablespoons sliced toasted almonds

*This recipe was tested with sucralose-based sugar substitute.

1. Combine yogurt, preserves, sugar substitute and vanilla in medium bowl.

2. Layer ½ cup yogurt mixture, ¼ cup strawberries, ¼ cup blueberries and ¼ cup yogurt mixture in each of four dessert dishes. Top each parfait with remaining ¼ cup strawberries and 1 tablespoon almonds. Serve immediately.

NOTES: These parfaits would also be delicious topped with low-fat granola. Or, try another flavor of preserves for a simple variation.

NUTRITIONAL INFORMATION

Calories **179**, Total Fat **3g**, Saturated Fat **1g**, Cholesterol **4mg**, Sodium **104mg**, Carbohydrates **33g**, Dietary Fiber **3g**, Protein **10g**

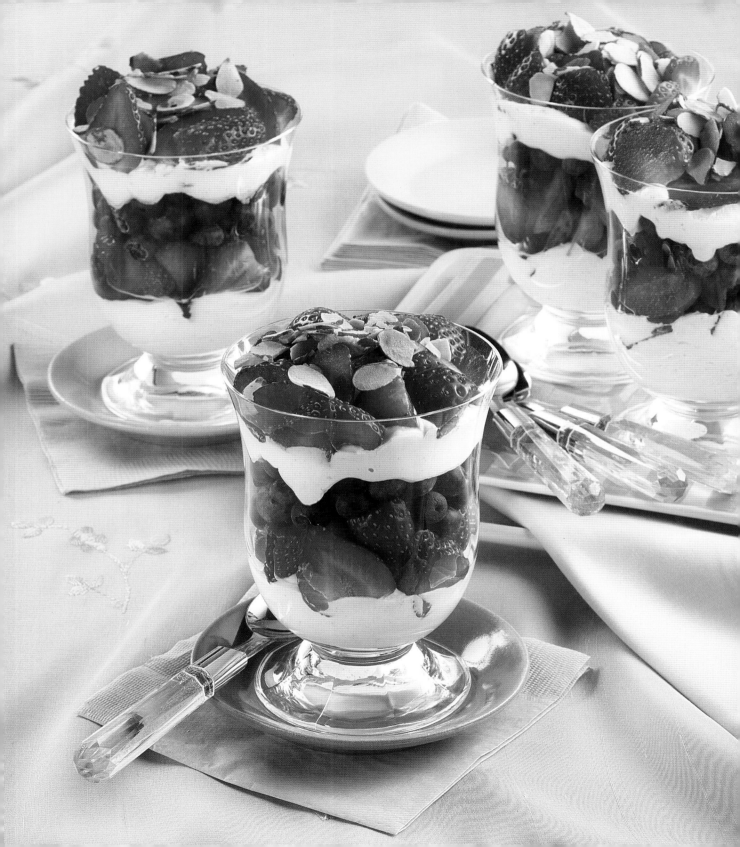

BREAKFAST QUINOA

Makes 2 servings

½ cup uncooked quinoa

1 cup water

1 tablespoon packed brown sugar

2 teaspoons maple syrup

½ teaspoon ground cinnamon

¼ cup golden raisins (optional)

Milk (optional)

Fresh raspberries and banana slices

1. Place quinoa in fine-mesh strainer; rinse well under cold running water. Transfer to small saucepan.

2. Stir in 1 cup water, brown sugar, maple syrup and cinnamon; bring to a boil over high heat. Reduce heat to low; cover and simmer 10 to 15 minutes or until quinoa is tender and water is absorbed. Add raisins, if desired, during last 5 minutes of cooking. Serve with milk, if desired; top with raspberries and bananas.

NUTRITIONAL INFORMATION

Calories **233**, Total Fat **3g**, Saturated Fat **1g**, Cholesterol **0mg**, Sodium **9mg**, Carbohydrates **47g**, Dietary Fiber **4g**, Protein **6g**

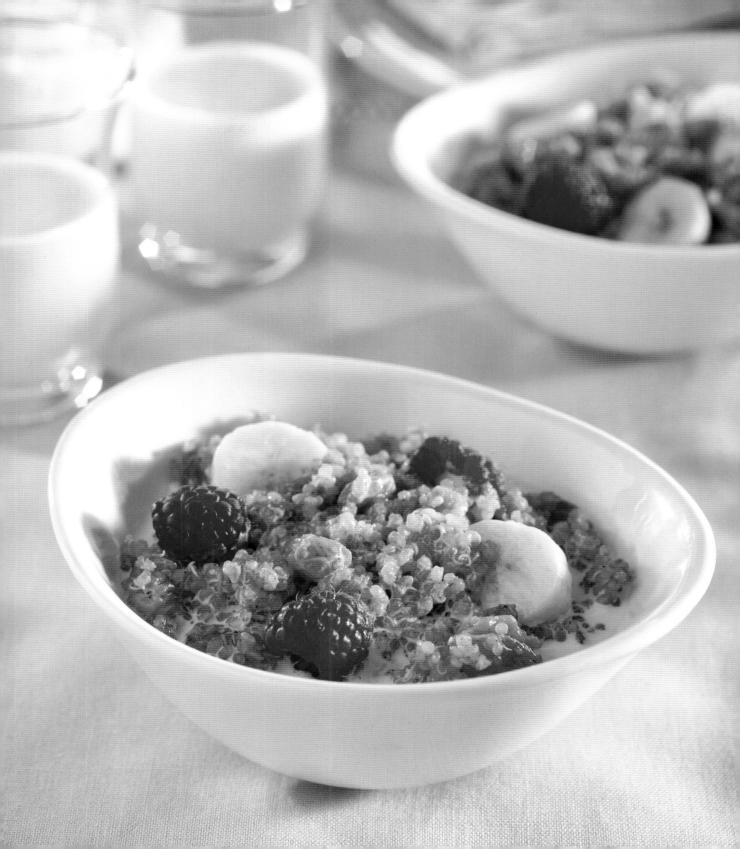

STRAWBERRY CINNAMON FRENCH TOAST

Makes 4 servings

1 egg

¼ cup fat-free (skim) milk

½ teaspoon vanilla

4 (1-inch-thick) diagonally-cut slices French bread (about 1 ounce each)

2 teaspoons reduced-fat margarine, softened

2 packets sugar substitute*

¼ teaspoon ground cinnamon

1 cup sliced fresh strawberries

This recipe was tested with sucralose-based sugar substitute.

1. Preheat oven to 450°F. Spray baking sheet with nonstick cooking spray.

2. Beat egg, milk and vanilla in shallow dish or pie plate. Lightly dip bread slices in egg mixture, coating completely. Place on prepared baking sheet.

3. Bake 15 minutes or until golden brown, turning halfway through baking time.

4. Meanwhile, combine margarine, sugar substitute and cinnamon in small bowl; stir until well blended. Spread mixture evenly over French toast; top with strawberries.

NUTRITIONAL INFORMATION

Calories **125**, Total Fat **3g**, Saturated Fat **1g**, Cholesterol **53mg**, Sodium **220mg**, Carbohydrates **19g**, Dietary Fiber **2g**, Protein **5g**

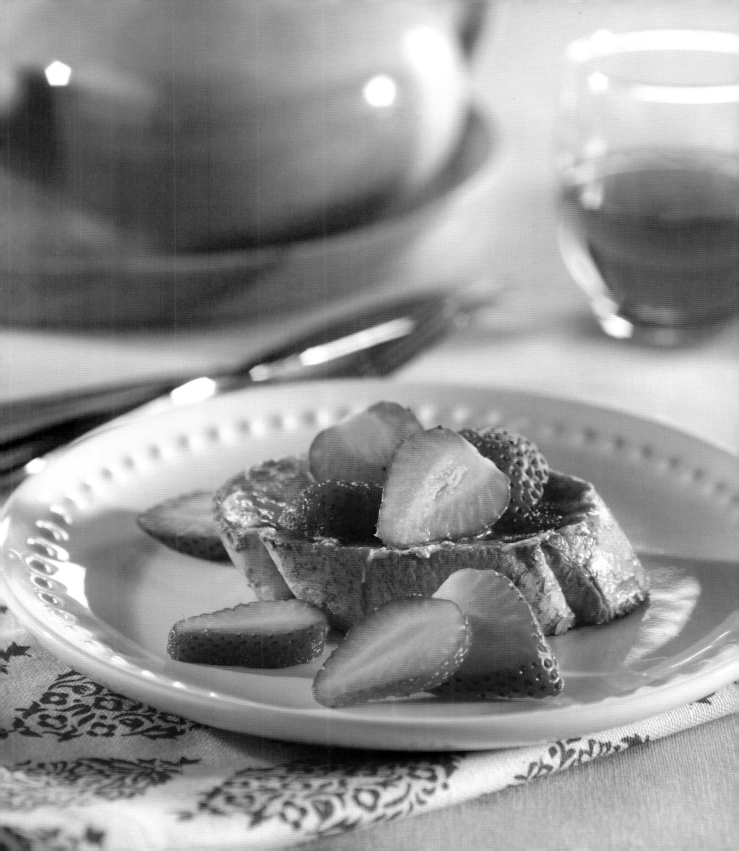

POTATO and PORK FRITTATA

Makes 4 servings

12 ounces (about 3 cups) frozen hash brown potatoes

1 teaspoon Cajun seasoning

4 egg whites

2 eggs

¼ cup low-fat (1%) milk

1 teaspoon dry mustard

¼ teaspoon black pepper

10 ounces (about 3 cups) frozen stir-fry vegetable blend

⅓ cup water

¾ cup chopped cooked lean pork

½ cup (2 ounces) shredded reduced-fat Cheddar cheese

1. Preheat oven to 400°F. Spray baking sheet with nonstick cooking spray. Spread potatoes on prepared baking sheet; sprinkle with Cajun seasoning. Bake 15 minutes or until hot. Remove from oven. *Reduce oven temperature to 350°F.*

2. Beat egg whites, eggs, milk, mustard and pepper in small bowl until well blended. Combine vegetables and water in medium ovenproof nonstick skillet; cook over medium heat 5 minutes or until vegetables are crisp-tender; drain. Add potatoes and pork to vegetables in skillet; stir gently. Add egg mixture; sprinkle with cheese. Cook over medium-low heat 5 minutes.

3. Bake 5 minutes or until egg mixture is set and cheese is melted. Cut into 4 wedges.

NUTRITIONAL INFORMATION

Calories **268**, Total Fat **11g**, Saturated Fat **5g**, Cholesterol **145mg**, Sodium **258mg**, Carbohydrates **20g**, Dietary Fiber **2g**, Protein **22g**

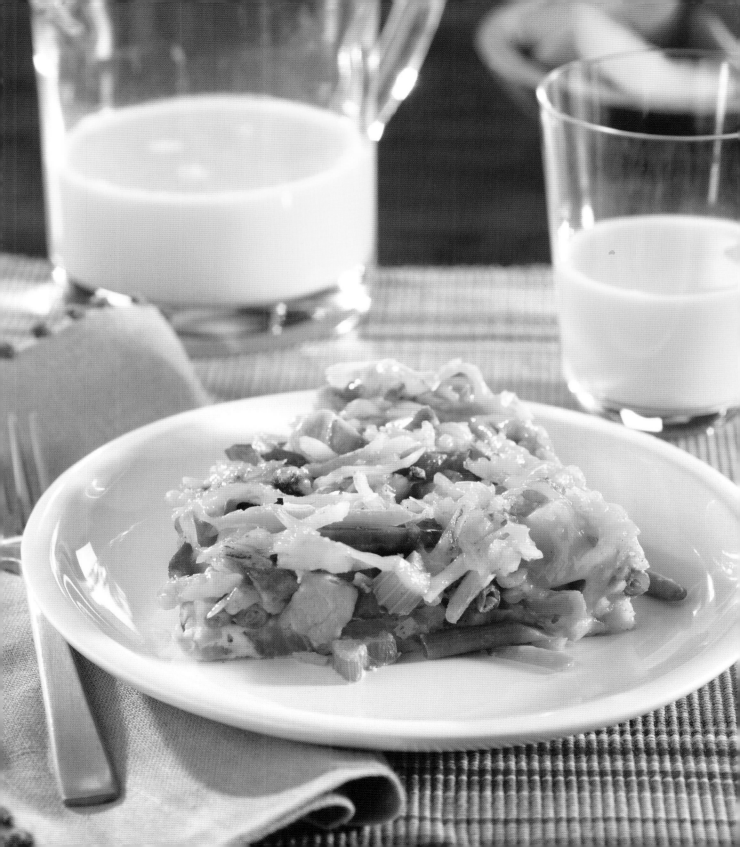

TROPICAL PARFAIT

Makes 4 servings

1½ cups orange or vanilla nonfat yogurt

1 can (11 ounces) mandarin orange segments in light syrup, drained and chopped

1 can (8 ounces) pineapple chunks in juice, drained

1 medium banana, sliced

2 tablespoons shredded coconut, toasted*

To toast coconut, spread in single layer in heavy-bottomed skillet. Cook and stir over medium heat 1 to 2 minutes or until lightly browned. Remove from skillet immediately. Cool before using.

1. Combine yogurt and oranges in medium bowl; mix well.

2. Spoon half of yogurt mixture into four serving bowls; top with pineapple. Spoon remaining yogurt mixture over pineapple; top with banana slices. Sprinkle with coconut. Serve immediately.

NUTRITIONAL INFORMATION

Calories **170**, Total Fat **1g**, Saturated Fat **1g**, Cholesterol **0mg**, Sodium **60mg**, Carbohydrates **40g**, Dietary Fiber **2g**, Protein **4g**

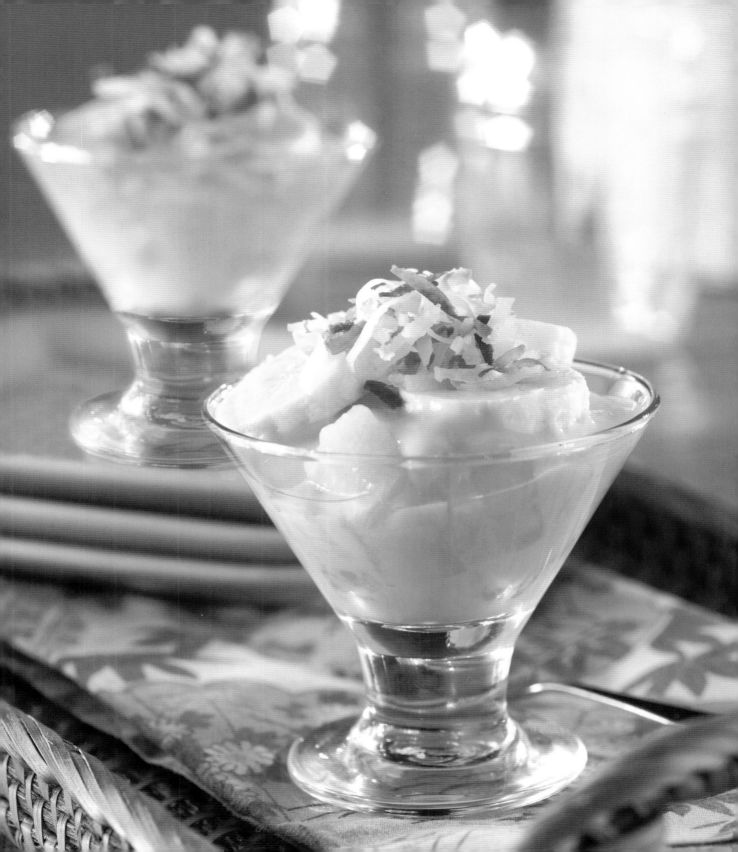

MEDITERRANEAN SCRAMBLE PITAS

Makes 4 servings

- 2 teaspoons canola oil, divided
- 1 cup sliced zucchini and/or yellow squash
- 1 cup diced green bell peppers
- 1 cup grape tomatoes, quartered
- ¼ teaspoon dried rosemary
- 12 small stuffed green olives, quartered
- ¼ cup finely chopped fresh Italian parsley
- 1 cup cholesterol-free egg substitute
- 2 multigrain pita bread rounds, halved and warmed
- 1 ounce reduced-fat feta cheese, crumbled

1. Heat 1 teaspoon oil in large nonstick skillet over medium-high heat. Add zucchini and bell peppers; cook 4 minutes or until crisp-tender. Add tomatoes and rosemary; cook 2 minutes, stirring frequently. Stir in olives and parsley. Place in medium bowl. Cover to keep warm.

2. Wipe out skillet with paper towel. Add remaining 1 teaspoon oil and heat over medium heat. Cook egg substitute until set, lifting edges to allow uncooked portion to flow underneath.

3. Fill each warmed pita half with equal amounts of eggs and feta. Top with vegetable mixture and remaining feta.

NUTRITIONAL INFORMATION

Calories **199**, Total Fat **7g**, Saturated Fat **1g**, Cholesterol **2mg**, Sodium **554mg**, Carbohydrates **26g**, Dietary Fiber **6g**, Protein **12g**

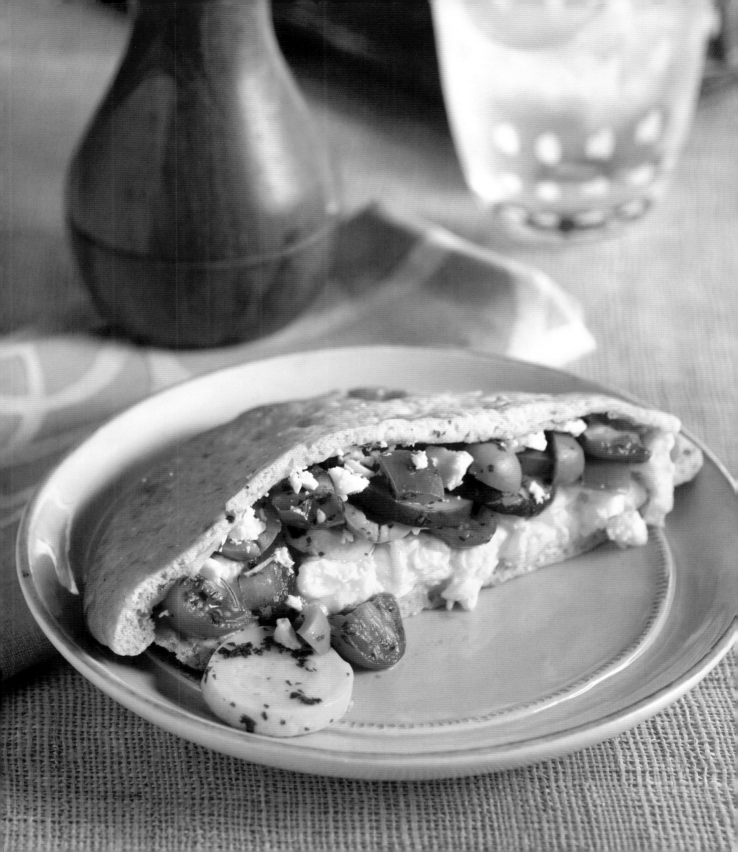

ZUCCHINI BREAD PANCAKES

Makes 3 servings (2 pancakes per serving)

1 medium zucchini, grated

¼ cup vanilla nonfat yogurt

1 egg

2 tablespoons fat-free (skim) milk

1 tablespoon vegetable oil

½ cup whole wheat flour

2 tablespoons packed brown sugar

1 teaspoon grated lemon peel, plus additional for garnish

1 teaspoon baking soda

½ teaspoon ground cinnamon

⅛ teaspoon ground nutmeg

Sugar-free maple syrup (optional)

1. Combine zucchini, yogurt, egg, milk and oil in large bowl; mix well. Add flour, brown sugar, 1 teaspoon lemon peel, baking soda, cinnamon and nutmeg; stir just until combined.

2. Heat large nonstick griddle or skillet over medium-low heat. Pour ¼ cupfuls of batter 2 inches apart onto griddle. Cook 3 minutes or until lightly browned and edges begin to bubble. Turn over; cook 3 minutes or until lightly browned. Repeat with remaining batter.

3. Serve with maple syrup, if desired. Garnish with additional lemon peel.

NUTRITIONAL INFORMATION

Calories **198**, Total Fat **7g**, Saturated Fat **1g**, Cholesterol **63mg**, Sodium **468mg**, Carbohydrates **29g**, Dietary Fiber **3g**, Protein **7g**

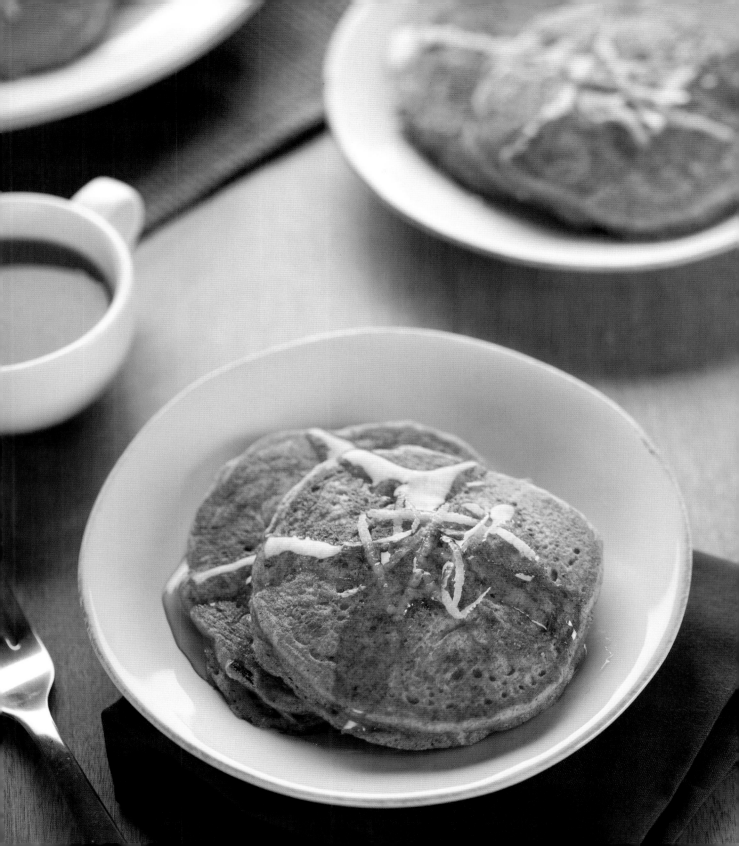

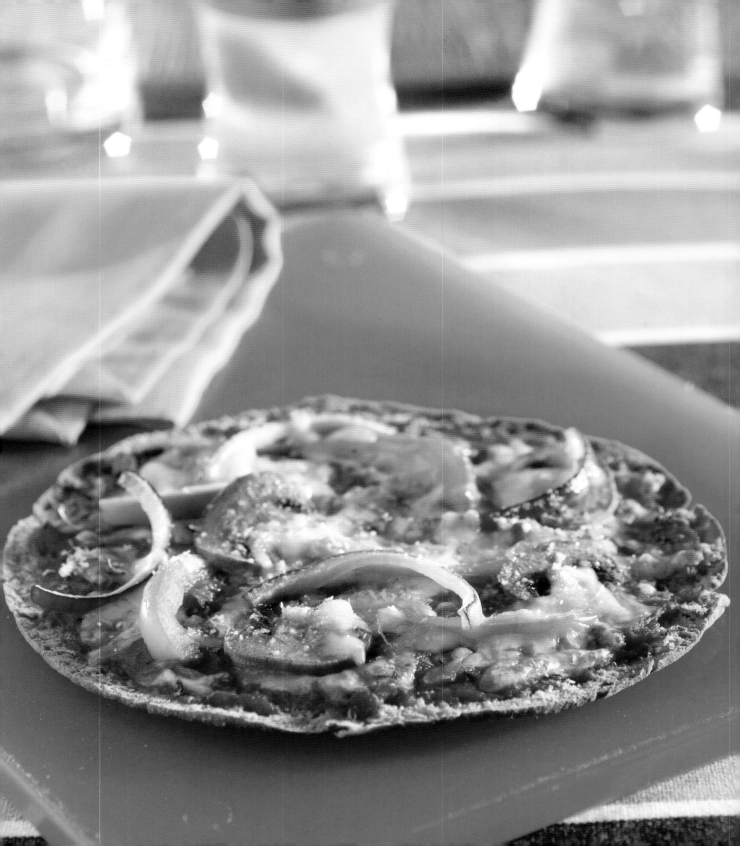

LUNCHES & LIGHTER FARE

VEGGIE PIZZA PITAS

Makes 4 servings

2 whole wheat pita bread rounds, cut in half horizontally (to make 4 rounds)

¼ cup pizza sauce

1 teaspoon dried basil

⅛ teaspoon red pepper flakes (optional)

1 cup sliced mushrooms

½ cup thinly sliced green bell pepper

½ cup thinly sliced red onion

1 cup (4 ounces) shredded part-skim mozzarella cheese

2 teaspoons grated Parmesan cheese

1. Preheat oven to 475°F.

2. Arrange pita rounds, rough sides up, in single layer on large nonstick baking sheet. Spread 1 tablespoon pizza sauce evenly over each round to within ¼ inch of edge. Sprinkle with basil and red pepper flakes, if desired. Top with mushrooms, bell pepper and onion. Sprinkle with mozzarella cheese.

3. Bake 5 minutes or until mozzarella cheese is melted. Sprinkle ½ teaspoon Parmesan cheese over each round.

NUTRITIONAL INFORMATION

Calories **113**, Total Fat **2g**, Saturated Fat **1g**, Cholesterol **6mg**, Sodium **402mg**, Carbohydrates **13g**, Dietary Fiber **2g**, Protein **11g**

WARM BLACKENED TUNA SALAD

Makes 4 servings

5 cups torn romaine lettuce

2 cups coarsely shredded red cabbage

2 medium yellow or green bell peppers, cut into strips

1½ cups sliced zucchini

⅓ cup water

¾ cup sliced onion

2 tablespoons balsamic vinegar

1½ teaspoons Dijon mustard

1 teaspoon canola or vegetable oil

½ teaspoon chicken bouillon granules

1 teaspoon onion powder

½ teaspoon garlic powder

½ teaspoon dried thyme

½ teaspoon ground red pepper

½ teaspoon black pepper

12 ounces fresh or thawed frozen tuna steaks, cut 1 inch thick

1. Preheat broiler. Spray broiler pan with nonstick cooking spray. Combine romaine, cabbage, bell peppers and zucchini in large bowl; set aside.

2. For dressing, bring water to a boil in small saucepan over high heat. Add onion slices; reduce heat to medium-low. Cover and simmer 4 to 5 minutes or until onion is tender. Add vinegar, mustard, oil and bouillon granules; cook and stir until heated through.

3. Combine onion powder, garlic powder, thyme, red pepper and black pepper in small bowl. Rub spice mixture onto both sides of tuna. Place tuna on broiler pan. Broil 4 inches from heat about 10 minutes or to desired doneness, turning once.

4. Divide vegetable mixture among four salad plates; slice tuna and arrange on top. Drizzle with dressing. Serve warm.

NUTRITIONAL INFORMATION

Calories **196**, Total Fat **6g**, Saturated Fat **1g**, Cholesterol **32mg**, Sodium **185mg**, Carbohydrates **13g**, Dietary Fiber **4g**, Protein **23g**

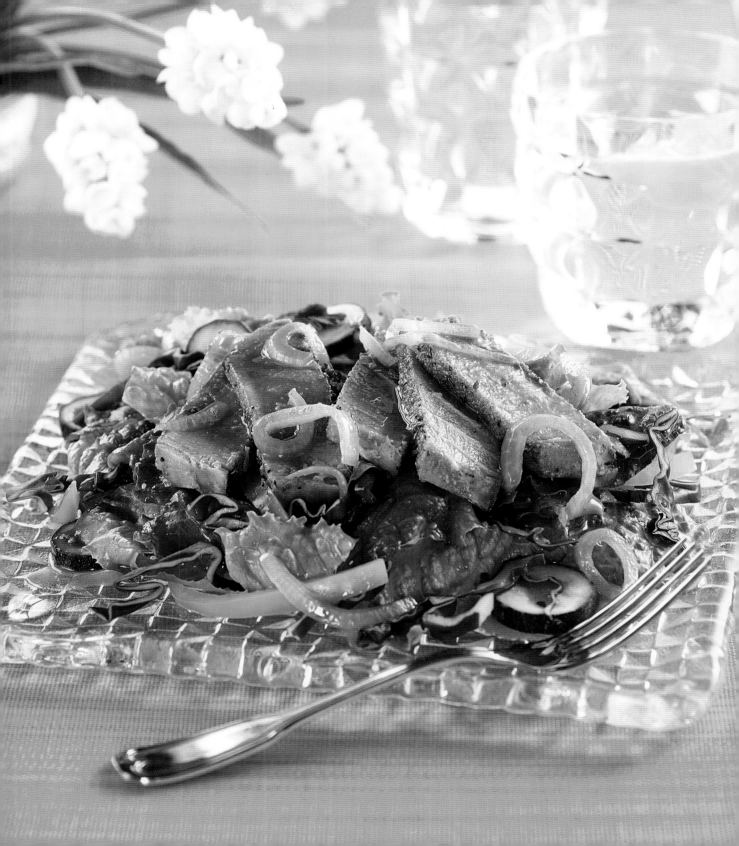

CHICKEN SALAD PITAS

Makes 4 servings

4 cups torn mixed spring greens

2 cups (about 8 ounces) chopped cooked chicken breast

½ cup chopped green bell pepper or poblano pepper

½ cup reduced-fat ranch salad dressing

4 whole wheat pita bread rounds, halved crosswise

Black pepper (optional)

1. Combine greens, chicken, bell pepper and salad dressing in large bowl; toss to coat. Microwave pita halves on HIGH 12 to 15 seconds.

2. Fill warmed pita halves evenly with salad mixture. Sprinkle with black pepper, if desired.

NUTRITIONAL INFORMATION

Calories **325**, Total Fat **4g**, Saturated Fat **1g**, Cholesterol **54mg**, Sodium **561mg**, Carbohydrates **44g**, Dietary Fiber **6g**, Protein **29g**

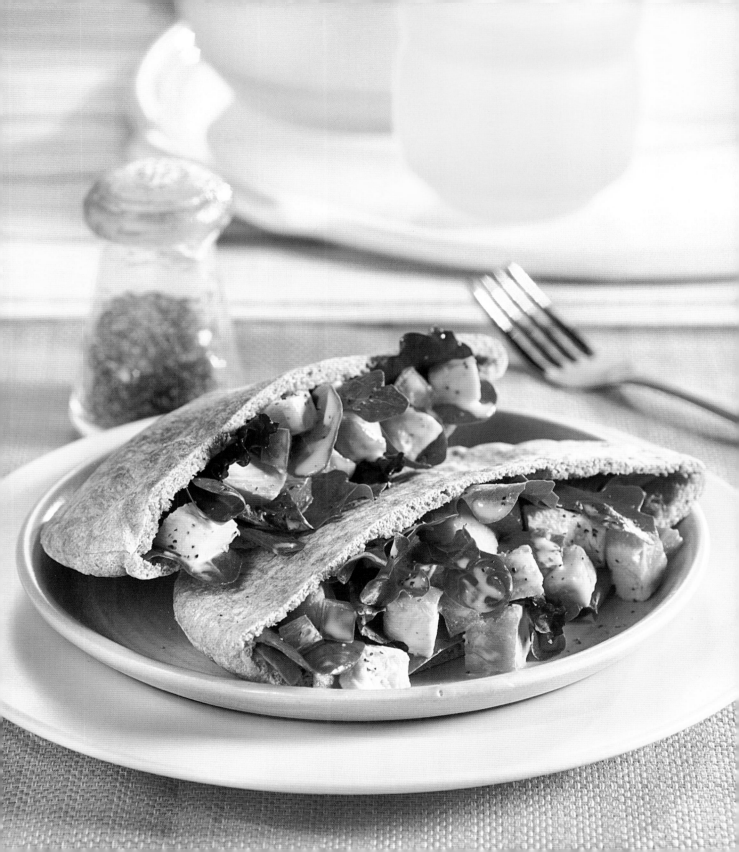

SAUSAGE AND CHEESE PIZZA

Makes 8 servings

1 can (about 14 ounces)
    refrigerated pizza crust dough

1 medium red onion, thinly sliced

4 ounces cooked turkey sausage
    breakfast links (5 to 6 links),
    thinly sliced

1 medium green bell pepper, thinly
    sliced

¾ cup pizza sauce

    Red pepper flakes (optional)

1 cup (4 ounces) shredded low-fat
    Monterey Jack or pizza cheese
    blend

1. Preheat oven to 425°F. Spray 15×10-inch jelly-roll pan with nonstick cooking spray. Unroll crust on pan; press to edges of pan. Bake about 6 minutes or until crust begins to brown.

2. Spray large nonstick skillet with cooking spray. Cook and stir onion over medium-high heat until tender. Add sausage and bell pepper to skillet. Cook and stir about 5 minutes or until bell pepper is crisp-tender.

3. Spread pizza sauce evenly over crust; top with sausage mixture. Sprinkle with red pepper flakes, if desired. Top with cheese.

4. Bake 7 to 10 minutes or until crust is golden brown and cheese is melted. Cut pizza into 8 pieces to serve.

NUTRITIONAL INFORMATION

Calories **212**, Total Fat **7g**, Saturated Fat **3g**, Cholesterol **19mg**, Sodium **618mg**, Carbohydrates **26g**, Dietary Fiber **1g**, Protein **11g**

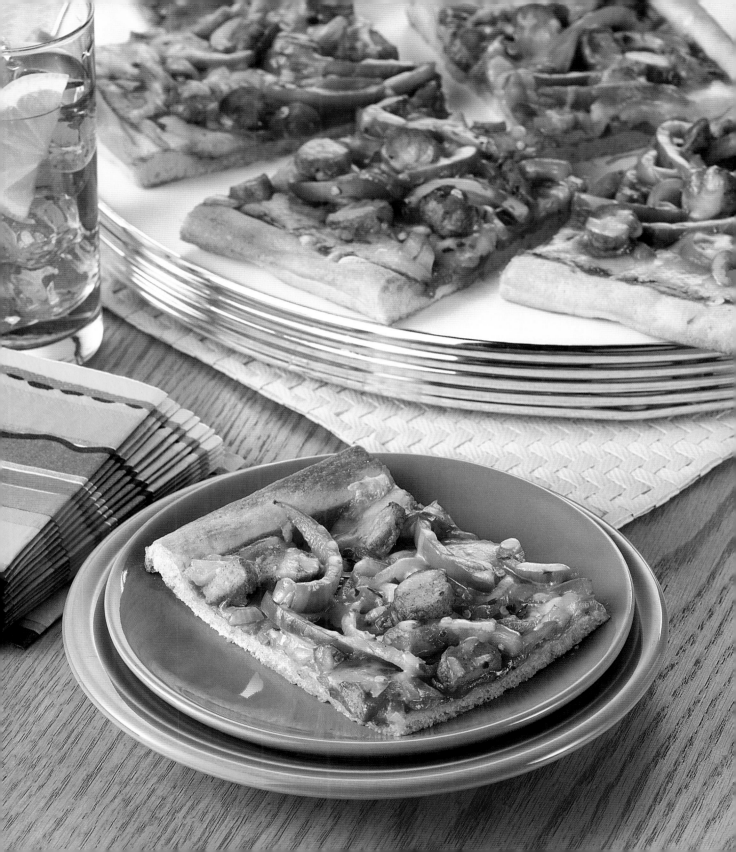

SPICY VEGETABLE QUESADILLAS

Makes 8 servings

1 small zucchini, chopped

½ cup chopped onion

½ cup chopped green bell pepper

2 cloves garlic, minced

½ teaspoon chili powder

½ teaspoon ground cumin

8 (6-inch) flour tortillas

1 cup (4 ounces) shredded reduced-fat Cheddar cheese

¼ cup chopped fresh cilantro

1. Spray large skillet with nonstick cooking spray; heat over medium heat. Add zucchini, onion, bell pepper, garlic, chili powder and cumin; cook and stir 3 to 4 minutes or until vegetables are crisp-tender.

2. Spoon vegetable mixture evenly over half of each tortilla. Sprinkle evenly with cheese and cilantro. Fold each tortilla in half.

3. Wipe skillet clean. Spray skillet with cooking spray. Add quesadillas; heat over medium heat 1 to 2 minutes per side or until lightly browned.

NUTRITIONAL INFORMATION

Calories **153**, Total Fat **4g**, Saturated Fat **1g**, Cholesterol **8mg**, Sodium **201mg**, Carbohydrates **23g**, Dietary Fiber **1g**, Protein **7g**

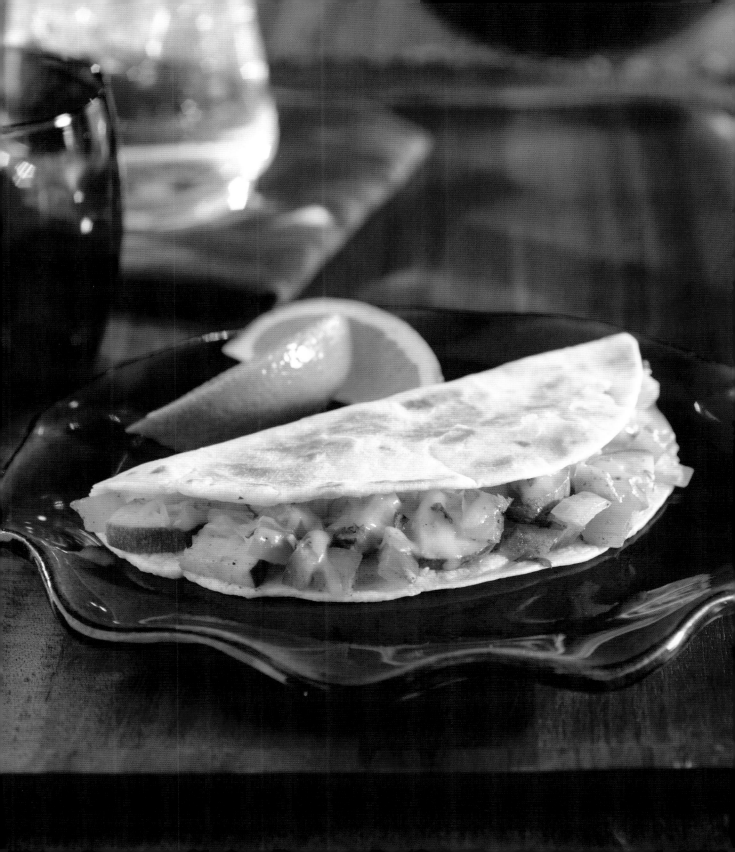

MEDITERRANEAN TUNA SANDWICHES

Makes 4 servings

1 can (12 ounces) solid white tuna packed in water, drained

¼ cup finely chopped red onion

¼ cup fat-free or reduced-fat mayonnaise

3 tablespoons chopped black olives, drained

1 tablespoon plus 1 teaspoon lemon juice

1 tablespoon chopped fresh mint (optional)

1 tablespoon olive oil

¼ teaspoon black pepper

⅛ teaspoon garlic powder (optional)

8 slices whole wheat bread

8 pieces romaine lettuce

8 thin slices tomato

1. Combine tuna, onion, mayonnaise, olives, lemon juice, mint, if desired, oil, pepper and garlic powder, if desired, in large bowl until blended.

2. Top each of 4 slices bread with tomato slice and lettuce leaf. Spoon ⅔ cup tuna mixture over each tomato slice. Top with remaining bread slices. Cut sandwiches in half to serve.

NUTRITIONAL INFORMATION

Calories **332**, Total Fat **12g**, Saturated Fat **2g**, Cholesterol **31mg**, Sodium **483mg**, Carbohydrates **27g**, Dietary Fiber **4g**, Protein **29g**

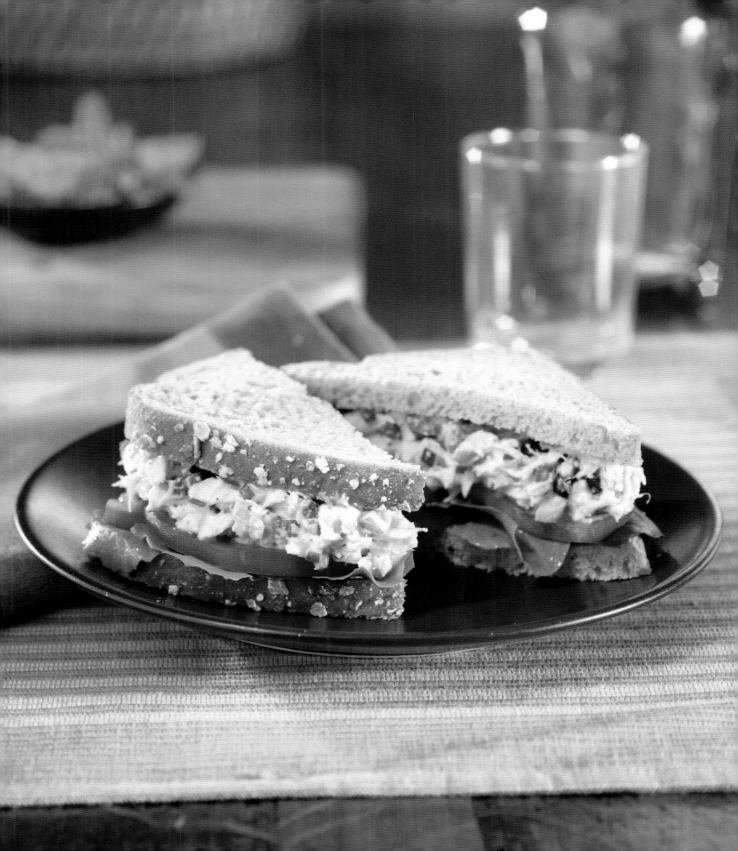

PIZZA-STUFFED POTATOES

Makes 4 servings

4 medium potatoes (about 7 ounces each)

¾ cup pizza sauce

⅛ teaspoon garlic powder

2 teaspoons grated Parmesan cheese

1 ounce turkey pepperoni slices (about 16), quartered

¾ cup (3 ounces) shredded part-skim mozzarella cheese

MICROWAVE DIRECTIONS

1. Poke potatoes with fork and heat in microwave on HIGH 5 to 7 minutes or until soft. Split potatoes open with a knife; mash insides lightly.

2. Top each potato with 3 tablespoons pizza sauce; mix lightly into potato.

3. Sprinkle potatoes evenly with garlic powder and Parmesan cheese. Top evenly with pepperoni and mozzarella cheese.

4. Return potatoes to microwave; cook on HIGH 1 minute or until cheese is melted.

NUTRITIONAL INFORMATION

Calories **258**, Total Fat **5g**, Saturated Fat **2g**, Cholesterol **23mg**, Sodium **547mg**, Carbohydrates **42g**, Dietary Fiber **5g**, Protein **13g**

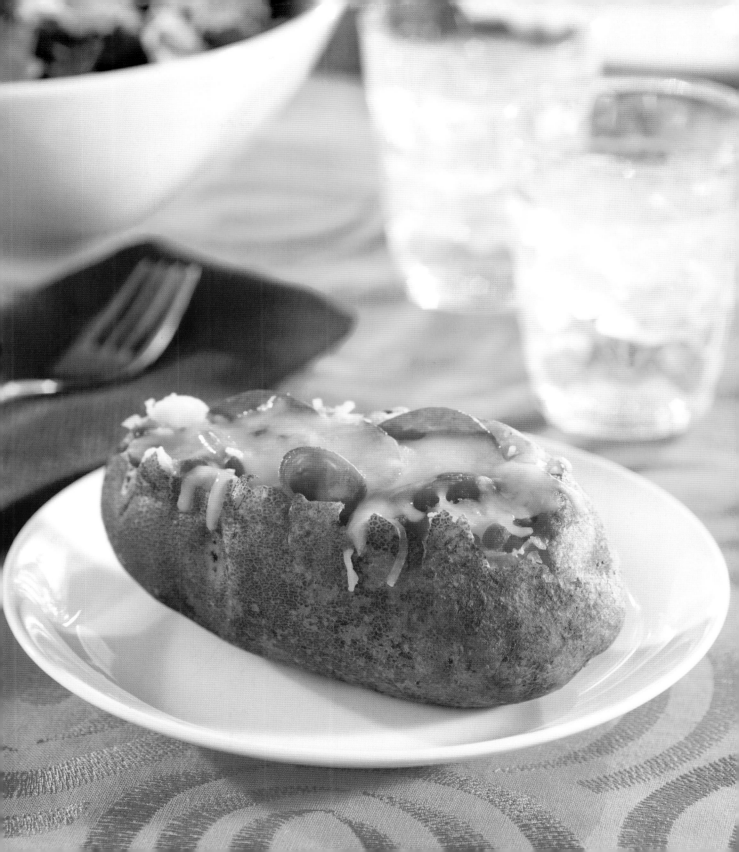

TURKEY & VEGGIE ROLL-UPS

Makes 2 servings

2 tablespoons hummus, any flavor

1 (8-inch) whole wheat tortilla

¼ cup sliced baby spinach

2 slices oven-roasted turkey breast (about 1 ounce)

¼ cup thinly sliced English cucumber

1 slice (1 ounce) reduced-fat Swiss cheese

¼ cup thinly sliced carrot

Spread hummus on tortilla to within 1 inch of edge. Layer with spinach, turkey, cucumber, cheese and carrots. Roll up tortilla and filling; cut into 4 pieces.

NUTRITIONAL INFORMATION

Calories **140**, Total Fat **4g**, Saturated Fat **1g**, Cholesterol **16mg**, Sodium **292mg**, Carbohydrates **14g**, Dietary Fiber **2g**, Protein **11g**

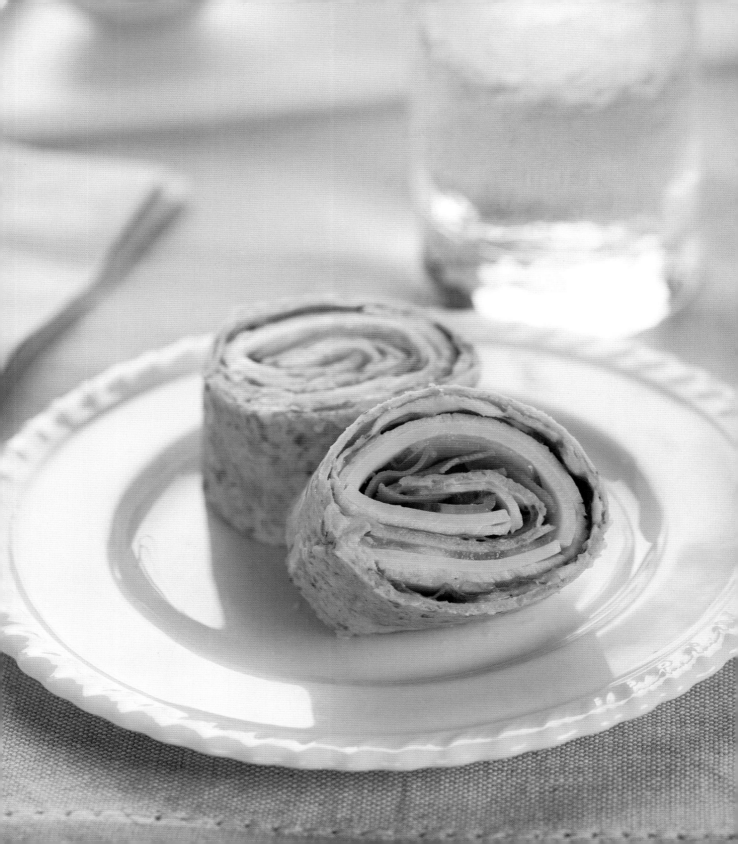

PEPPER PITA PIZZAS

Makes 4 servings

1 teaspoon olive oil

1 medium onion, thinly sliced

1 medium red bell pepper, cut into thin strips

1 medium green bell pepper, cut into thin strips

4 cloves garlic, minced

2 tablespoons minced fresh basil *or* 2 teaspoons dried basil

1 tablespoon minced fresh oregano *or* 1 teaspoon dried oregano

2 Italian plum tomatoes, coarsely chopped

4 (6-inch) pita bread rounds

1 cup (4 ounces) shredded reduced-fat Monterey Jack cheese

1. Preheat oven to 425°F. Heat oil in medium nonstick skillet over medium heat until hot. Add onion, bell peppers, garlic, basil and oregano. Partially cover; cook 5 minutes or until tender, stirring occasionally. Add tomatoes. Partially cover and cook 3 minutes.

2. Place pita rounds on baking sheet. Divide tomato mixture evenly among pitas; top each pita with ¼ cup cheese. Bake 5 minutes or until cheese is melted.

NUTRITIONAL INFORMATION

Calories **302**, Total Fat **7g**, Saturated Fat **3g**, Cholesterol **20mg**, Sodium **552mg**, Carbohydrates **44g**, Dietary Fiber **2g**, Protein **16g**

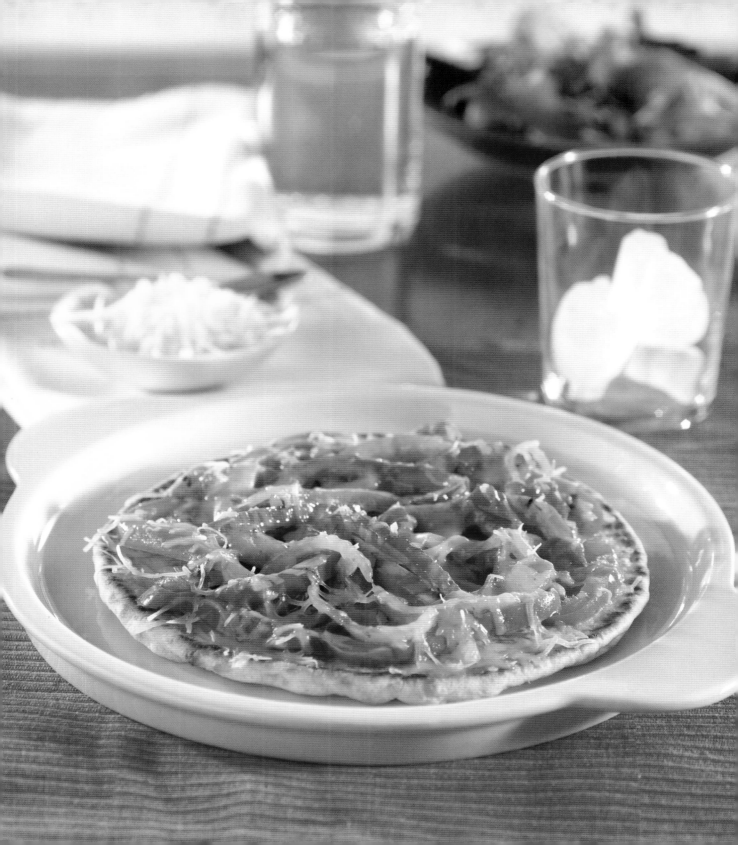

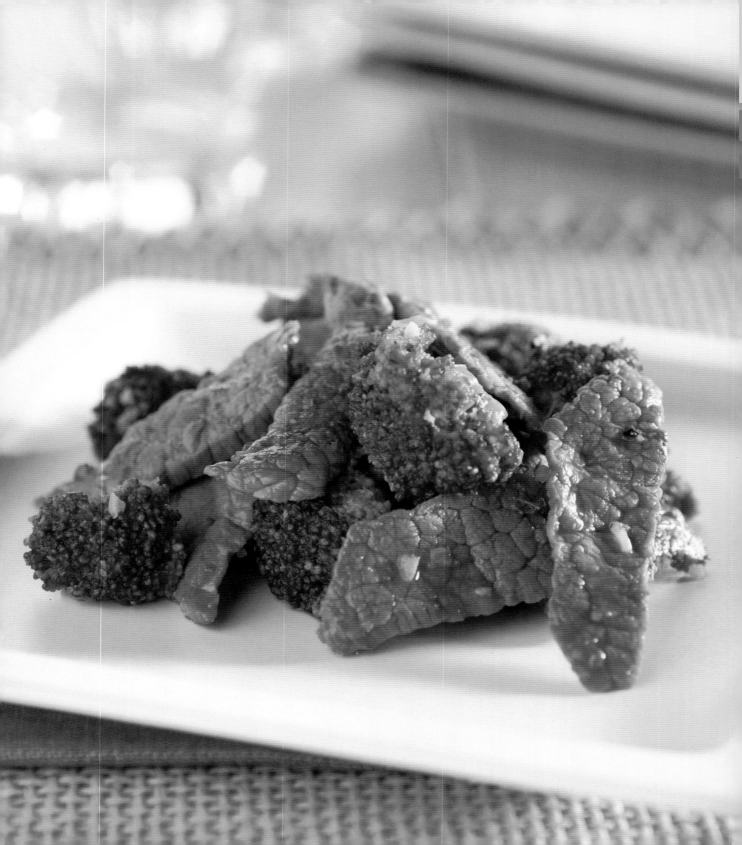

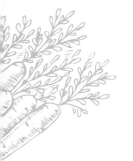

MAIN DISHES

GARLIC BEEF

Makes 4 servings

1 teaspoon dark sesame oil

1 pound beef eye of round, trimmed, cut into thin strips

1 package (10 ounces) frozen chopped broccoli

1 tablespoon minced garlic

1 tablespoon light soy sauce

¼ teaspoon black pepper

Heat oil in 12-inch nonstick skillet over high heat. Add beef, broccoli, garlic, soy sauce and pepper. Cook, stirring occasionally, 15 minutes or until beef is cooked through.

NUTRITIONAL INFORMATION

Calories **214**, Total Fat **9g**, Saturated Fat **3g**, Cholesterol **42mg**, Sodium **320mg**, Carbohydrates **6g**, Dietary Fiber **2g**, Protein **27g**

BAKED COD WITH TOMATOES AND OLIVES

Makes 4 servings

1 pound cod fillets (about 4 fillets), cut into 2-inch pieces

Salt and black pepper

1 can (about 14 ounces) diced Italian-style tomatoes

2 tablespoons chopped pitted black olives

1 teaspoon minced garlic

2 tablespoons chopped fresh parsley

1. Preheat oven to 400°F. Spray 13×9-inch baking dish with nonstick cooking spray. Arrange cod fillets in dish; season with salt and pepper.

2. Combine tomatoes, olives and garlic in medium bowl. Spoon over fish.

3. Bake 20 minutes or until fish begins to flake when tested with fork. Sprinkle with parsley.

SERVING SUGGESTION: For a great accompaniment to this dish, spread French bread with softened butter, sprinkle with paprika and oregano, and broil until lightly toasted.

NUTRITIONAL INFORMATION

Calories **121**, Total Fat **1g**, Saturated Fat **1g**, Cholesterol **48mg**, Sodium **574mg**, Carbohydrates **5g**, Dietary Fiber **1g**, Protein **21g**

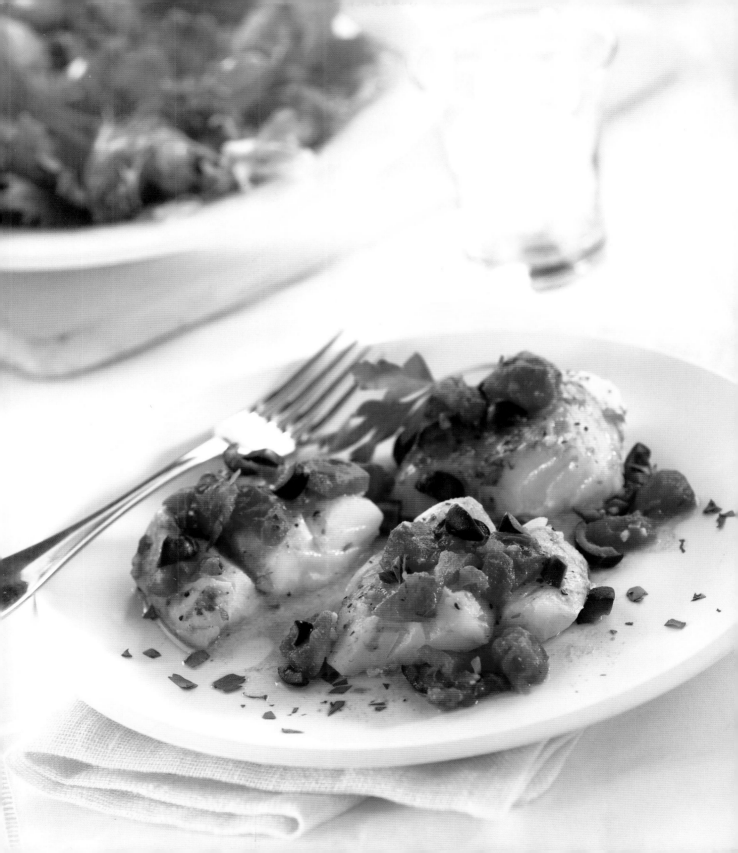

FAJITA-SEASONED GRILLED CHICKEN

Makes 2 servings

2 boneless skinless chicken breasts (about 4 ounces each)

1 bunch green onions, ends trimmed

1 tablespoon olive oil

2 teaspoons fajita seasoning mix

1. Prepare grill for direct cooking.

2. Brush chicken and green onions with oil. Sprinkle both sides of chicken breasts with seasoning mix. Grill chicken and green onions 6 to 8 minutes or until chicken is no longer pink in center.

3. Serve chicken with green onions.

FAJITA-SEASONED GRILLED CHICKEN BOWL: Prepare chicken as directed above. Slice chicken and serve on plate or bowl with cooked corn, kidney beans, cut-up tomatoes, chopped red onions, diced avocados and rice pilaf. Garnish with lime wedges, if desired.

NUTRITIONAL INFORMATION

Calories **176**, Total Fat **8g**, Saturated Fat **1g**, Cholesterol **43mg**, Sodium **186mg**, Carbohydrates **8g**, Dietary Fiber **2g**, Protein **19g**

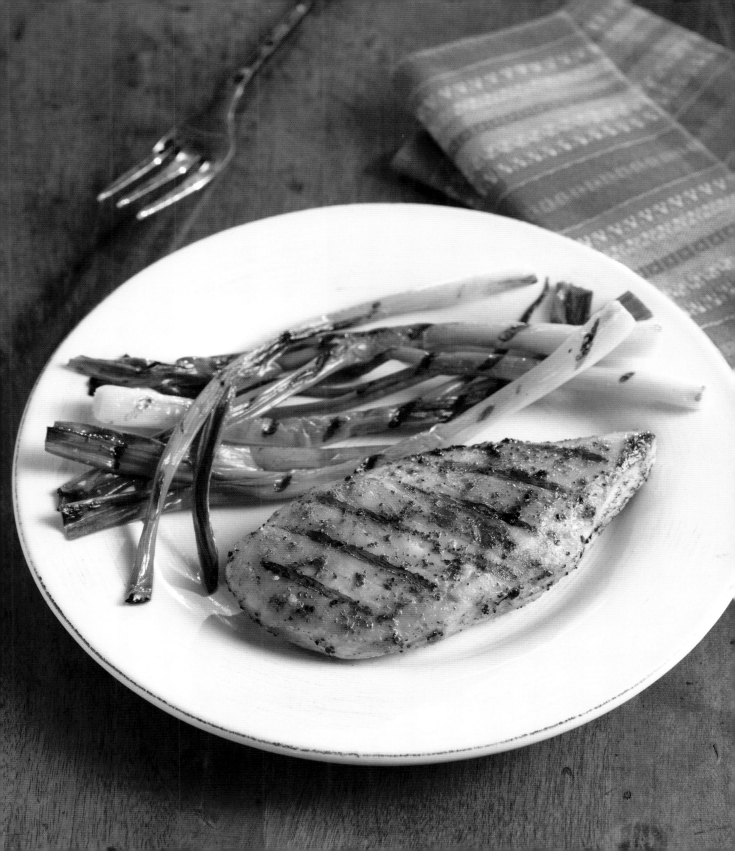

PORK CHOPS AND STUFFING SKILLET CASSEROLE

Makes 4 servings

4 thin bone-in pork chops (1 pound)

¼ teaspoon dried thyme

¼ teaspoon paprika

⅛ teaspoon salt

¼ pound 50% less fat bulk pork sausage

2 cups corn bread stuffing mix

1¼ cups water

1 cup frozen diced green bell peppers, thawed

⅛ to ¼ teaspoon poultry seasoning (optional)

1. Preheat oven to 350°F. Sprinkle one side of pork chops with thyme, paprika and salt. Spray large ovenproof skillet with nonstick cooking spray; heat over medium-high heat. Add pork, seasoned side down; cook 2 minutes. Remove to plate; keep warm.

2. Add sausage to skillet; cook 6 to 8 minutes or until no longer pink, stirring to break up meat. Remove from heat; stir in stuffing mix, water, bell peppers and poultry seasoning, if desired, until just blended.

3. Arrange pork, seasoned side up, over stuffing mixture. Cover; bake 15 minutes or until pork is no longer pink in center. Let stand 5 minutes before serving.

NUTRITIONAL INFORMATION

Calories **305**, Total Fat **14g**, Saturated Fat **5g**, Cholesterol **92mg**, Sodium **499mg**, Carbohydrates **13g**, Dietary Fiber **3g**, Protein **28g**

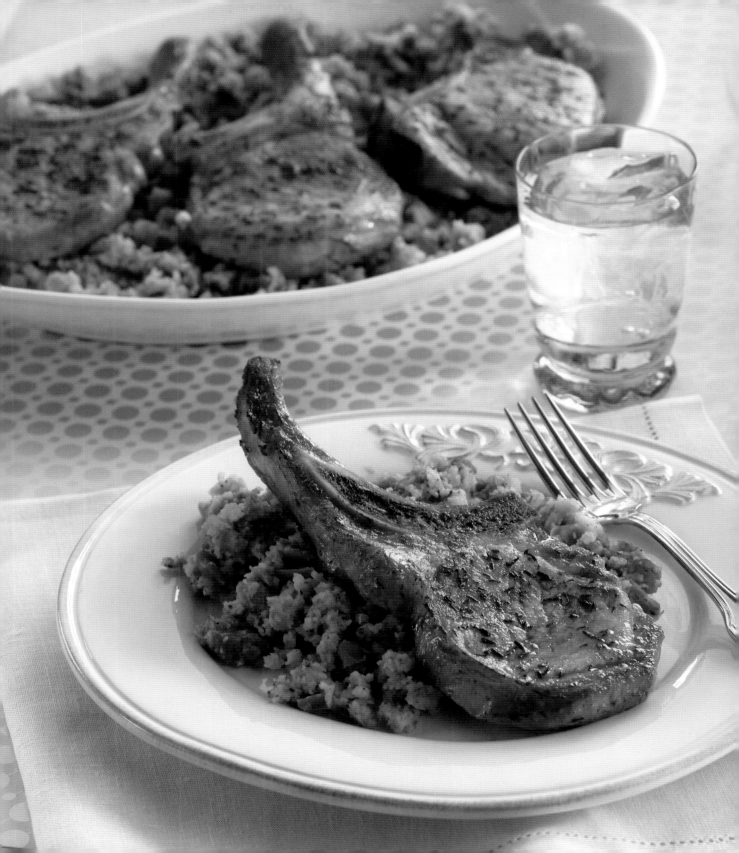

WHOLE WHEAT PENNE PASTA WITH SUMMER VEGETABLES

Makes 4 servings

6 ounces uncooked whole wheat penne pasta (about 2 cups)

2 teaspoons olive oil

2 cloves garlic, minced

1½ cups chopped fresh broccoli

1 medium zucchini, chopped (about 1¼ cups)

½ medium yellow bell pepper, chopped (about ¾ cup)

8 ounces (about 1½ cups) cherry or grape tomatoes, halved

3 ounces (about 1 cup) mushrooms, sliced

½ teaspoon dried oregano

¾ cup crumbled reduced-fat feta cheese

1. Cook pasta according to package directions, omitting any salt or fat. Drain and keep warm.

2. Heat oil in large nonstick skillet over medium-high heat. Add garlic, broccoli, zucchini and bell pepper. Cook and stir about 2 minutes or until vegetables just begin to soften.

3. Add tomatoes, mushrooms and oregano; mix well. Reduce heat to medium and cook and stir about 8 minutes or until vegetables are tender and tomatoes release their juices.

4. Mix vegetables with pasta. Toss with feta cheese.

NUTRITIONAL INFORMATION

Calories **264**, Total Fat **7g**, Saturated Fat **3g**, Cholesterol **8mg**, Sodium **374mg**, Carbohydrates **41g**, Dietary Fiber **7g**, Protein **15g**

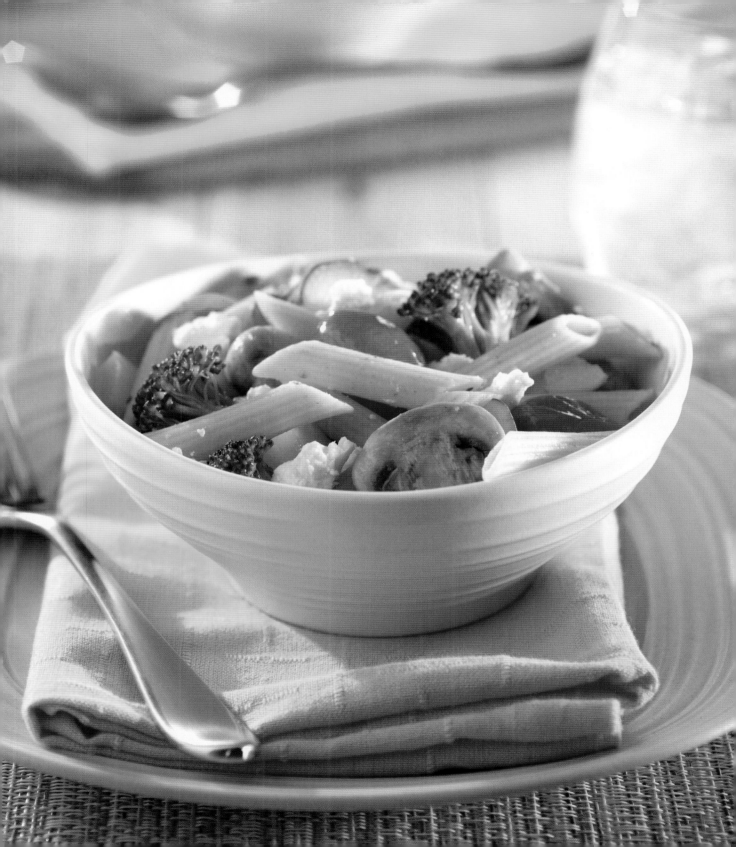

TILAPIA WITH SPINACH AND FETA

Makes 2 servings

1 teaspoon olive oil

1 clove garlic, minced

4 cups baby spinach

2 skinless tilapia fillets or other mild white fish (4 ounces each)

¼ teaspoon black pepper

2 ounces reduced-fat feta cheese, cut into 2 (3-inch) pieces

1. Preheat oven to 350°F. Spray baking sheet with nonstick cooking spray.

2. Heat oil in medium skillet over medium-low heat. Add garlic; cook and stir 30 seconds. Add spinach; cook just until wilted, stirring occasionally.

3. Arrange tilapia on prepared baking sheet; sprinkle with pepper. Place one piece of cheese on each fillet; top with spinach mixture.

4. Fold one end of each fillet up and over filling; secure with toothpick. Repeat with opposite end of each fillet.

5. Bake 20 minutes or until fish begins to flake when tested with fork.

NUTRITIONAL INFORMATION

Calories **193**, Total Fat **9g**, Saturated Fat **3g**, Cholesterol **10mg**, Sodium **531mg**, Carbohydrates **3g**, Dietary Fiber **1g**, Protein **26g**

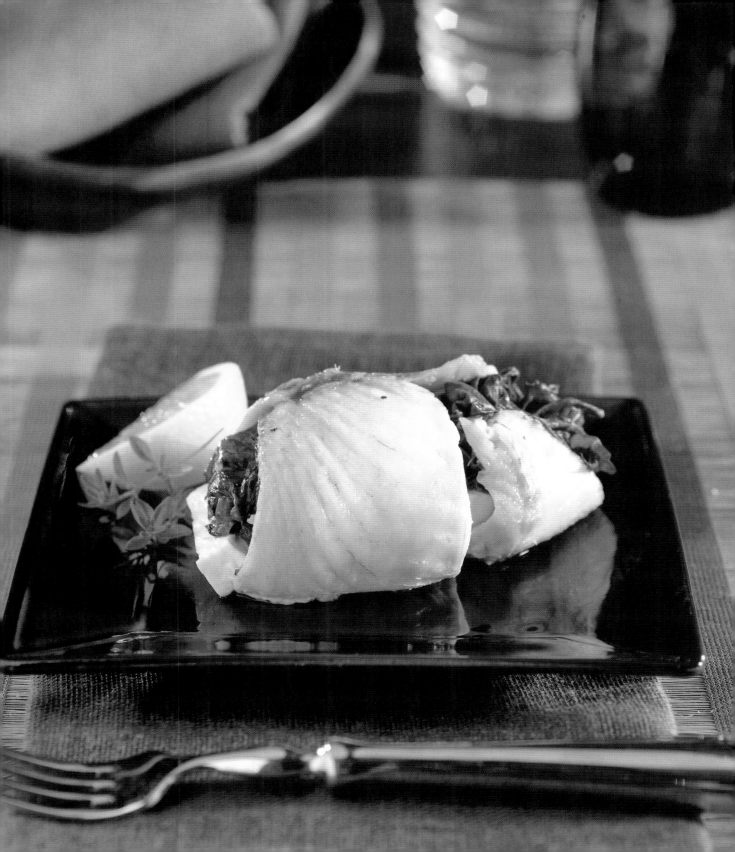

EASY CHEESY HAM AND VEGGIE RICE CASSEROLE

Makes 4 servings

- 1 bag (3½ ounces) boil-in-bag brown rice
- 2 cups broccoli florets
- 1 cup (3 ounces) matchstick-size carrot pieces
- 6 ounces lean, reduced-sodium ham, diced

- 2 ounces Swiss cheese, broken into small pieces
- 3 ounces reduced-fat sharp Cheddar cheese, shredded
- 1 tablespoon reduced-fat margarine
- ⅛ teaspoon ground red pepper

1. Cook rice in large saucepan according to package directions, omitting salt and fat. Remove rice packet when cooked; reserve water.

2. Add broccoli and carrots to water in saucepan, bring to a boil, reduce heat, cover and simmer 3 minutes or until broccoli is crisp-tender.

3. Drain vegetables and return to saucepan. Stir in rice. Heat over medium-low heat. Add ham, Swiss cheese, one third of the Cheddar cheese, margarine and red pepper; stir gently. Sprinkle evenly with remaining Cheddar cheese; cover and cook 3 minutes or until cheese melts.

NUTRITIONAL INFORMATION

Calories **283**, Total Fat **12g**, Saturated Fat **6g**, Cholesterol **48mg**, Sodium **616mg**, Carbohydrates **26g**, Dietary Fiber **2g**, Protein **19g**

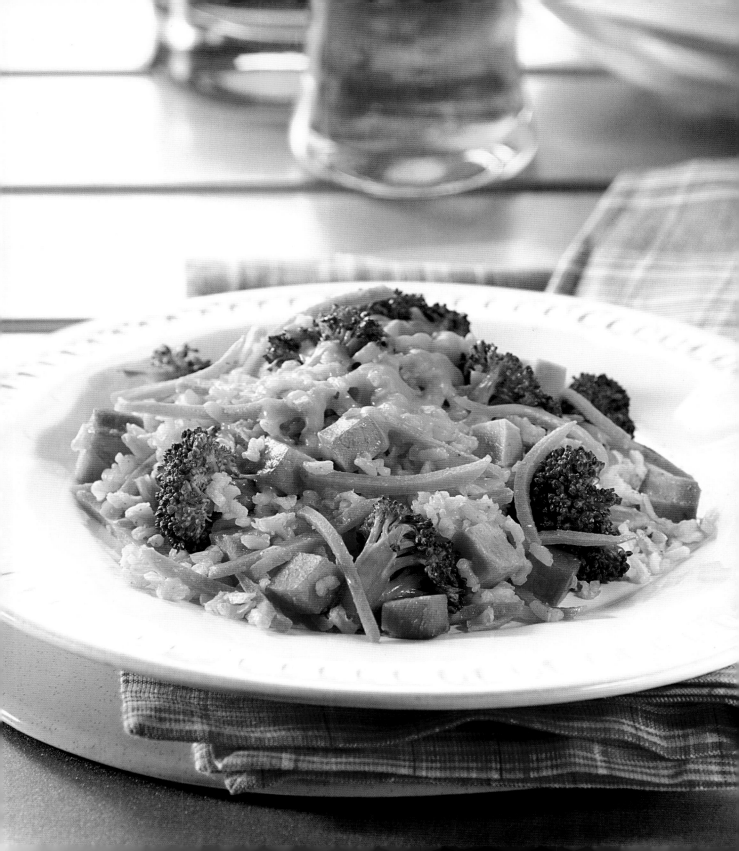

SPANISH-STYLE PORK WITH MANGO SALSA

Makes 4 servings

2 teaspoons canola oil

¾ cup coarsely chopped onion

2 cloves garlic, minced

¾ pound pork tenderloin, cut into 1-inch cubes

1 teaspoon ground cinnamon

1 teaspoon ground cumin

1 teaspoon dried oregano

½ teaspoon ground coriander

¼ teaspoon salt

1 medium mango, peeled and cut into bite-size pieces (about 1½ cups)

1 cup chunky salsa

2 cups cooked brown rice

2 tablespoons slivered almonds, toasted (optional)

1. Heat oil in large nonstick skillet over medium-high heat. Add onion; cook and stir 4 minutes or until tender. Add garlic; cook and stir 30 seconds. Add pork, cinnamon, cumin, oregano, coriander and salt; cook and stir 5 to 6 minutes or until pork is well browned on all sides.

2. Reduce heat to medium-low. Stir in mango and salsa. Cover and cook 3 to 4 minutes or until heated through. Serve over rice. Sprinkle with almonds, if desired.

NUTRITIONAL INFORMATION

Calories **309**, Total Fat **5g**, Saturated Fat **1g**, Cholesterol **55mg**, Sodium **510mg**, Carbohydrates **43g**, Dietary Fiber **4g**, Protein **21g**

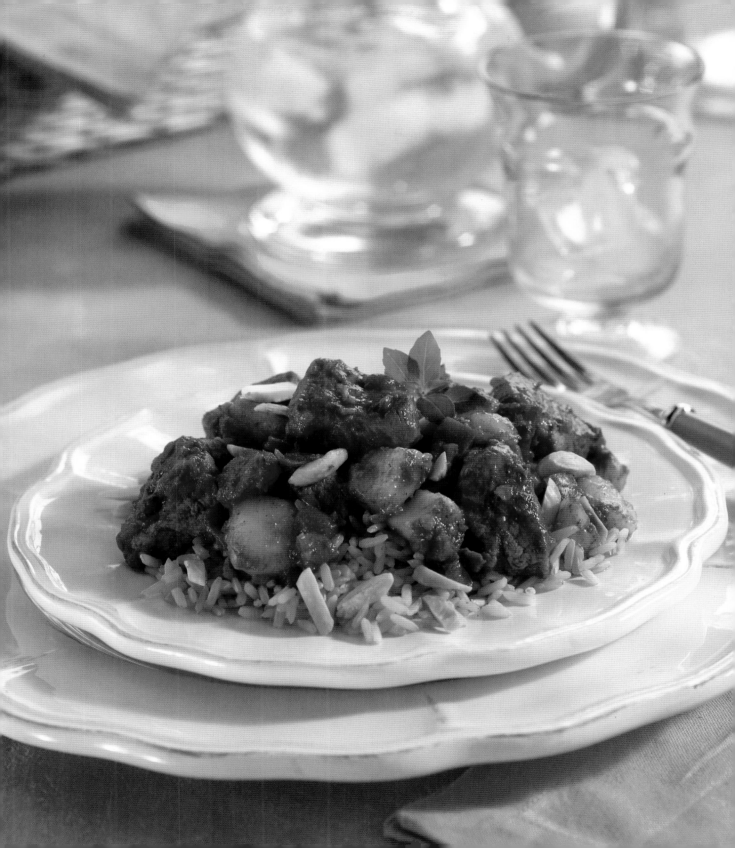

PAN-SEARED HALIBUT STEAKS WITH AVOCADO SALSA

Makes 4 servings

4 tablespoons chipotle salsa, divided

½ teaspoon salt, divided

4 small (4 to 5 ounces) *or* 2 large (8 to 10 ounces) halibut steaks, cut ¾ inch thick

½ cup diced tomato

½ ripe avocado, diced

2 tablespoons chopped fresh cilantro (optional)

Lime wedges (optional)

1. Combine 2 tablespoons salsa and ¼ teaspoon salt in small bowl; spread over both sides of halibut.

2. Heat large nonstick skillet over medium heat until hot. Add halibut; cook 4 to 5 minutes per side or until fish is opaque in center.

3. Meanwhile, combine remaining 2 tablespoons salsa, ¼ teaspoon salt, tomato, avocado and cilantro, if desired, in small bowl. Mix well and spoon over cooked fish. Garnish with lime wedges.

NUTRITIONAL INFORMATION

Calories **169**, Total Fat **7g**, Saturated Fat **1g**, Cholesterol **36mg**, Sodium **476mg**, Carbohydrates **2g**, Dietary Fiber **4g**, Protein **25g**

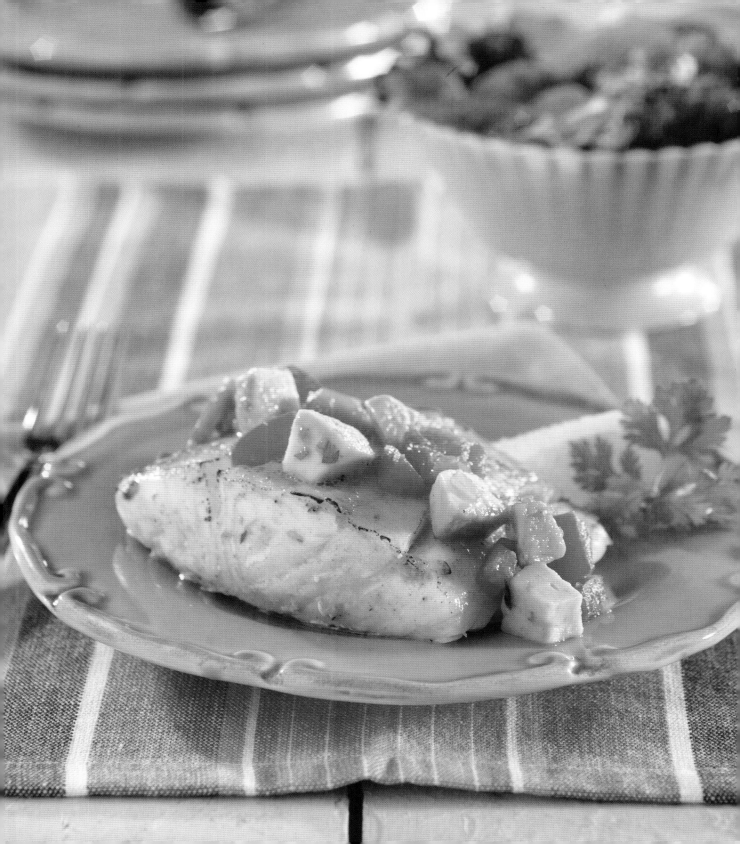

HERBED CHICKEN AND PASTA WITH SPANISH OLIVES

Makes 4 servings

- 4 ounces uncooked rotini pasta or rice
- 12 ounces boneless skinless chicken breasts, cut into bite-size pieces
- ½ teaspoon dried rosemary
- ¼ teaspoon dried thyme
- ¼ teaspoon red pepper flakes
- 4 cloves garlic, minced
- 1 cup grape tomatoes, quartered
- 3 ounces Spanish stuffed olives, halved lengthwise (about ½ cup)
- 2 tablespoons chopped fresh parsley
- 1½ cups packed baby spinach (1½ ounces), coarsely chopped
- 2 tablespoons extra virgin olive oil
- ⅛ teaspoon salt

1. Cook pasta according to package directions; drain and return to saucepan.

2. Meanwhile, spray large skillet with nonstick cooking spray and heat over medium-high heat. Cook and stir chicken, rosemary, thyme and red pepper flakes 2 minutes or until chicken is slightly pink in center. Add garlic; cook and stir 15 seconds. Stir in tomatoes, olives and parsley; cook until heated through.

3. Add chicken mixture, spinach, oil and salt to pasta; toss until spinach begins to wilt.

NUTRITIONAL INFORMATION

Calories **310**, Total Fat **11g**, Saturated Fat **1.5g**, Cholesterol **60mg**, Sodium **510mg**, Carbohydrates **28g**, Dietary Fiber **1g**, Protein **24g**

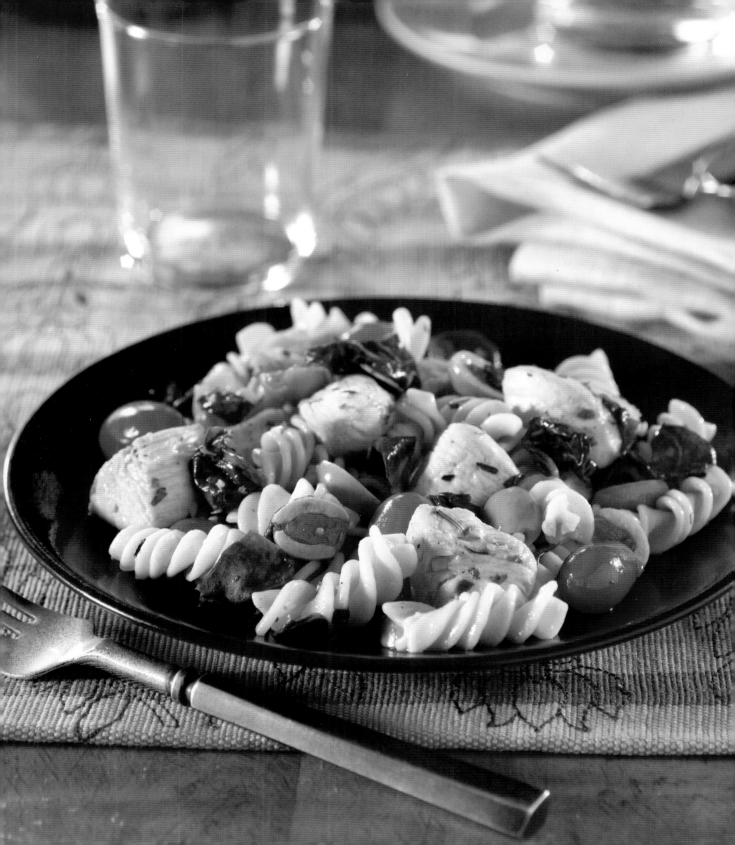

MINI MEATLOAVES

Makes 6 servings

3 tablespoons ketchup

1 tablespoon balsamic vinegar

1 tablespoon olive oil

1½ cups finely chopped onion

1½ cups finely chopped mushrooms

1½ cups chopped baby spinach

1½ pounds extra lean ground sirloin

¾ cup old-fashioned oats

2 egg whites

½ teaspoon salt

½ teaspoon black pepper

1. Preheat oven to 375°F. Spray six mini (4¼×2½-inch) loaf pans with nonstick cooking spray. Whisk ketchup and vinegar in small bowl until smooth and well blended; set aside.

2. Heat oil in large skillet over medium heat. Add onion, mushrooms and spinach; cook and stir 8 minutes or until tender. Remove to large bowl. Let stand until cool enough to handle.

3. Add beef, oats, egg whites, salt and pepper to vegetables; mix well. Divide mixture evenly among prepared pans. Brush half of ketchup mixture evenly over loaves.

4. Bake 15 minutes. Brush with remaining ketchup mixture. Bake 5 minutes or until cooked through (160°F).

NUTRITIONAL INFORMATION

Calories **270**, Total Fat **11g**, Saturated Fat **3g**, Cholesterol **62mg**, Sodium **362mg**, Carbohydrates **14g**, Dietary Fiber **2g**, Protein **28g**

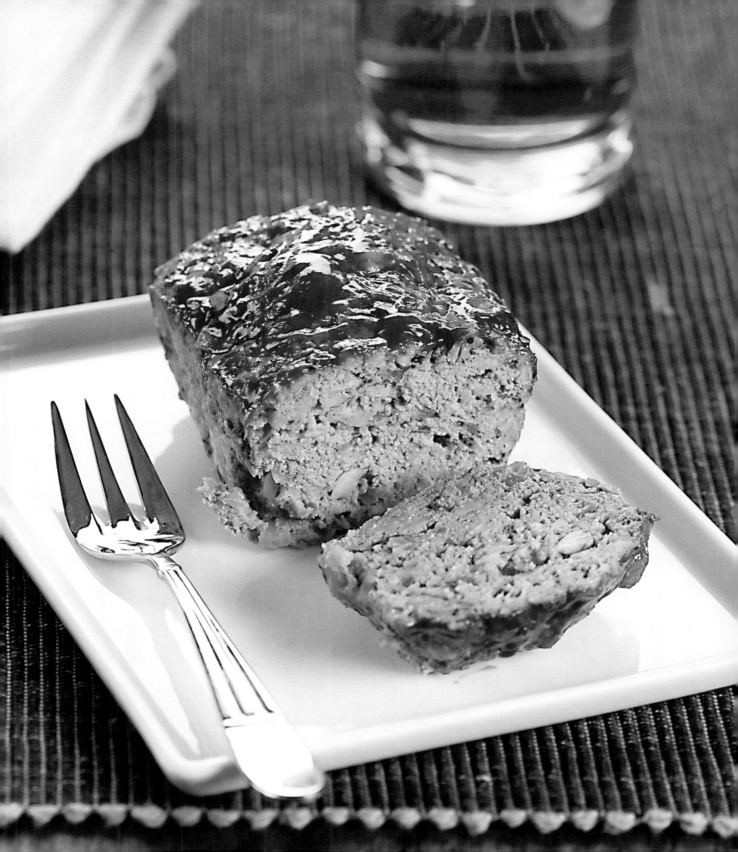

QUICK AND EASY SAUTÉED CHICKEN

Makes 4 servings

4 boneless skinless chicken breasts (4 ounces each)

1 teaspoon paprika (preferably smoked)

1 teaspoon dried thyme

½ teaspoon garlic salt

⅛ teaspoon ground red pepper

2 teaspoons olive oil

1. Place chicken breasts between sheets of waxed paper or plastic wrap; pound to even ½-inch thickness. Combine paprika, thyme, garlic salt and red pepper in small bowl; rub over both sides of chicken.

2. Heat oil in large nonstick skillet over medium heat. Add chicken; cook 4 to 5 minutes per side or until chicken is no longer pink in center. Pour any juices from skillet over chicken.

NUTRITIONAL INFORMATION

Calories **147**, Total Fat **4g**, Saturated Fat **1g**, Cholesterol **66mg**, Sodium **242mg**, Carbohydrates **1g**, Dietary Fiber **1g**, Protein **26g**

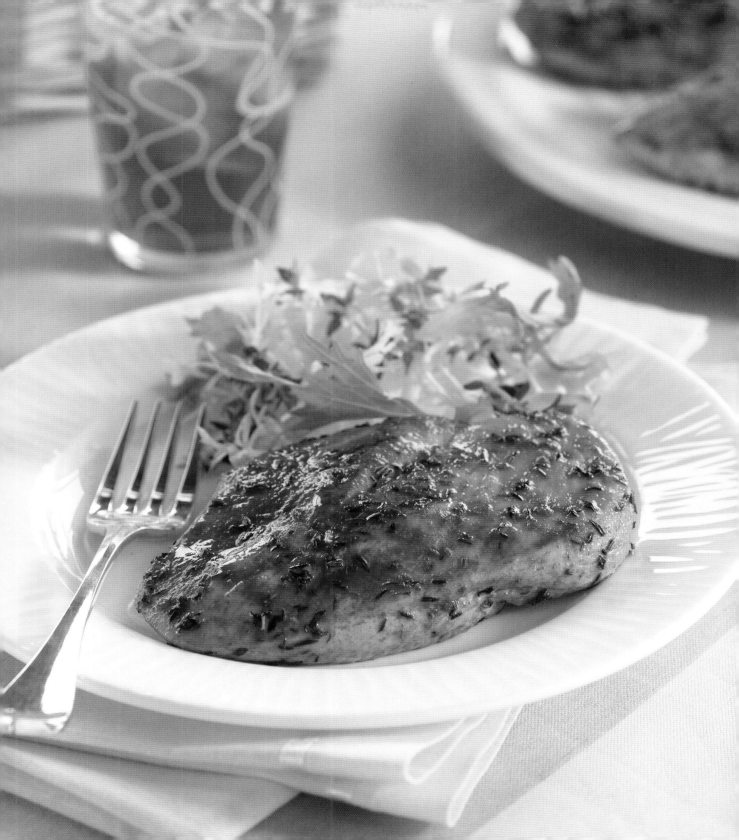

PORK AND PLUM KABOBS

Makes 4 servings

¾ pound boneless pork loin chops (1 inch thick), trimmed and cut into 1-inch pieces

1½ teaspoons ground cumin

½ teaspoon ground cinnamon

¼ teaspoon salt

¼ teaspoon garlic powder

¼ teaspoon ground red pepper

¼ cup sliced green onions

¼ cup raspberry fruit spread

1 tablespoon orange juice

3 plums or nectarines, pitted and cut into wedges

1. Place pork in large resealable food storage bag. Combine cumin, cinnamon, salt, garlic powder and red pepper in small bowl; pour over pork. Seal bag; shake to coat meat with spices.

2. Combine green onions, fruit spread and orange juice in small bowl; set aside.

3. Prepare grill for direct cooking. Alternately thread pork and plum wedges onto eight skewers.* Grill kabobs over medium heat 12 to 14 minutes or until meat is cooked through, turning once. Brush frequently with raspberry mixture during last 5 minutes of grilling.

If using wood skewers, soak in warm water 30 minutes to prevent burning.

SERVING SUGGESTION: A crisp, cool salad makes a great accompaniment to these sweet grilled kabobs.

NUTRITIONAL INFORMATION

Calories **191**, Total Fat **5g**, Saturated Fat **2g**, Cholesterol **53mg**, Sodium **183mg**, Carbohydrates **17g**, Dietary Fiber **1g**, Protein **19g**

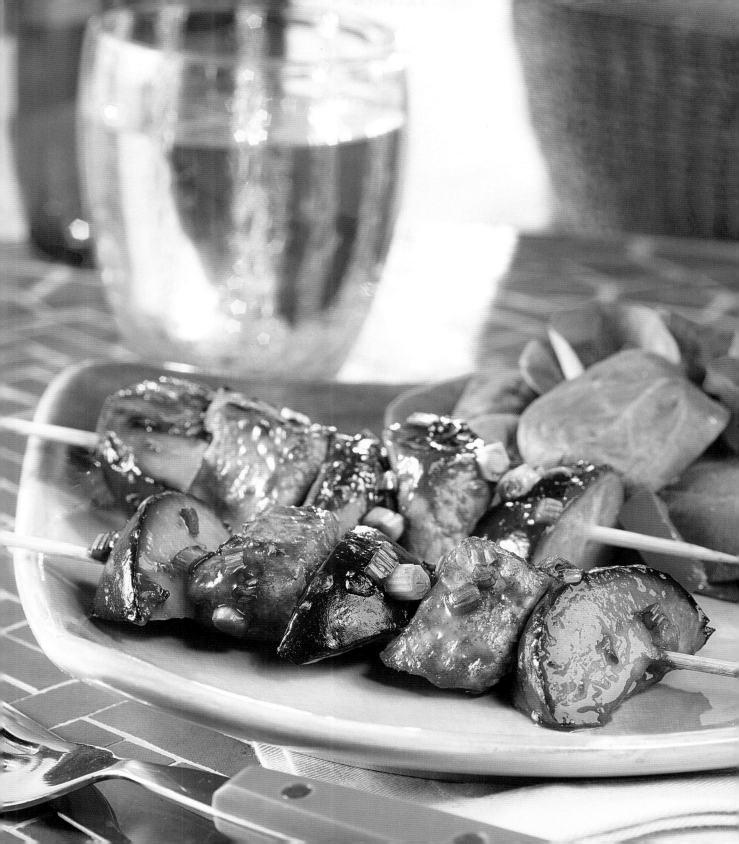

SALMON WITH DILL-MUSTARD SAUCE

Makes 4 servings

2 tablespoons fresh lemon juice

2 tablespoons fresh lime juice

4 salmon fillets (4 ounces each)

¼ cup fat-free mayonnaise

1 tablespoon Dijon mustard

1 tablespoon chopped fresh dill sprigs, plus additional for garnish

1. Combine lemon juice and lime juice in glass baking dish. Rinse salmon; pat dry. Place salmon in baking dish; turn to coat evenly. Marinate 10 minutes, turning once.

2. Stir mayonnaise, mustard and 1 tablespoon dill in small bowl until well blended.

3. Preheat broiler. Spray rack of broiler pan with nonstick cooking spray. Remove salmon from marinade; pat dry. Place on rack.

4. Broil 4 inches from heat source 3 to 4 minutes per side or until salmon begins to flake when tested with fork.

5. Place salmon on serving plates. Spoon evenly with sauce. Garnish with additional dill.

NUTRITIONAL INFORMATION

Calories **220**, Total Fat **12g**, Saturated Fat **3g**, Cholesterol **74mg**, Sodium **260mg**, Carbohydrates **3g**, Dietary Fiber **1g**, Protein **23g**

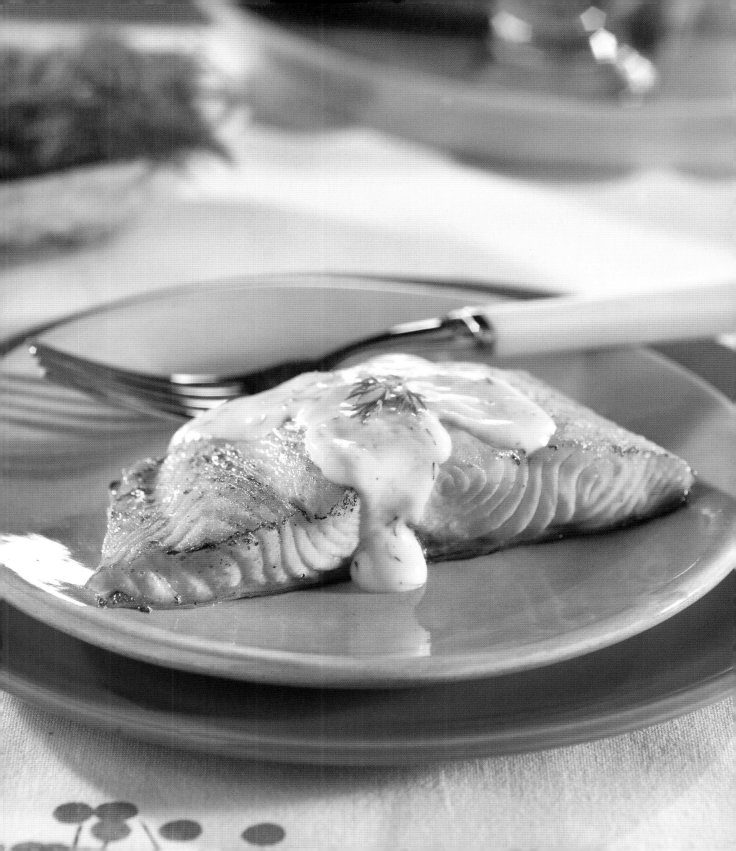

BEEF WITH SWEET PEPPERS AND EGGPLANT

Makes 4 servings

1 ounce pine nuts (about 3 tablespoons plus 1 teaspoon) or slivered almonds (about ¼ cup)

¾ pound lean ground beef

1 cup chopped yellow onion

⅓ medium eggplant (about 8 ounces), peeled and cubed

1 cup chopped red bell pepper

½ cup water

1 can (8 ounces) tomato sauce with herbs

¾ teaspoon ground cinnamon

¼ teaspoon ground allspice

1 cup uncooked instant rice

½ teaspoon salt

1. Heat 12-inch nonstick skillet over medium-high heat until hot. Add pine nuts; cook, stirring constantly, 2 minutes or until pine nuts begin to lightly brown. Remove to plate; set aside.

2. Spray same skillet with nonstick cooking spray. Add beef and onions; cook and stir about 4 minutes or until no longer pink. Add eggplant and bell pepper; coat lightly with cooking spray. Cook and stir 4 minutes or until eggplant is crisp-tender.

3. Add water; stir to blend. Add tomato sauce, cinnamon and allspice. Bring to a boil. Reduce heat. Cover tightly; simmer 10 minutes or until eggplant is tender and mixture has thickened slightly.

4. Meanwhile, cook rice according to package directions, omitting salt and fat.

5. Remove beef mixture from heat; stir salt and pine nuts into mixture. Cover tightly; let stand 5 minutes. Serve beef mixture over rice.

NUTRITIONAL INFORMATION

Calories **324**, Total Fat **10g**, Saturated Fat **2g**, Cholesterol **50mg**, Sodium **646mg**, Carbohydrates **37g**, Dietary Fiber **6g**, Protein **23g**

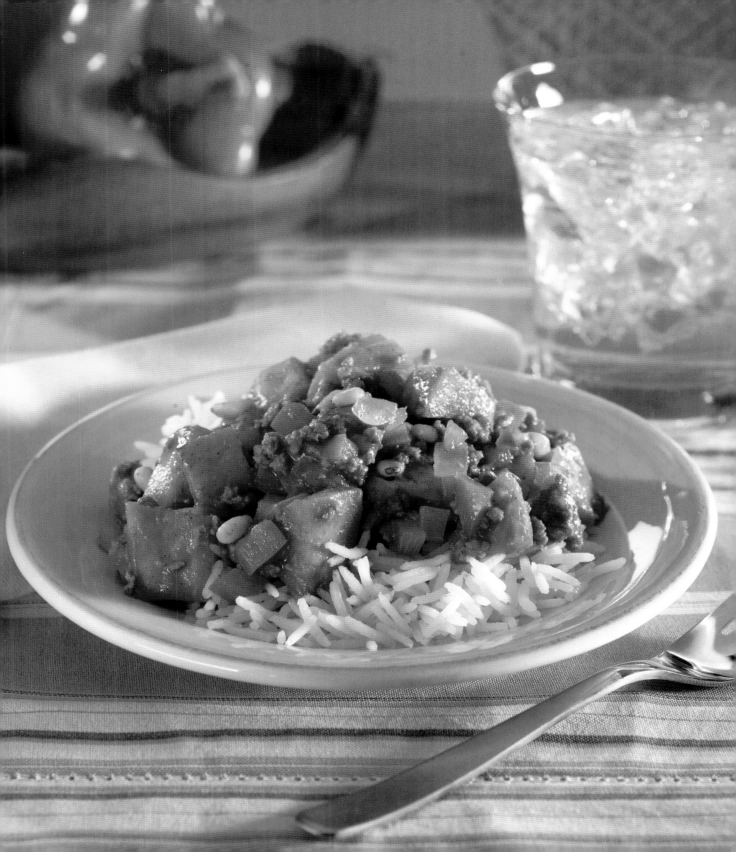

EASY SEAFOOD STIR-FRY

Makes 4 servings

1 package (1 ounce) dried black Chinese mushrooms*

½ cup fat-free reduced-sodium chicken broth

2 tablespoons dry sherry

1 tablespoon reduced-sodium soy sauce

4½ teaspoons cornstarch

1 teaspoon vegetable oil, divided

8 ounces bay scallops or halved sea scallops

4 ounces medium raw shrimp, peeled and deveined

2 cloves garlic, minced

6 ounces (2 cups) fresh snow peas, cut diagonally into halves

2 cups hot cooked rice

¼ cup thinly sliced green onions

Or substitute 1½ cups sliced fresh mushrooms and omit step 1.

1. Place mushrooms in medium bowl; cover with warm water. Soak 20 to 40 minutes or until soft. Drain and squeeze out excess water. Cut off and discard stems; cut caps into thin slices.

2. Whisk broth, sherry, soy sauce and cornstarch in small bowl until smooth.

3. Heat ½ teaspoon oil in wok or large nonstick skillet over medium heat. Add scallops, shrimp and garlic; stir-fry 3 minutes or until seafood is opaque. Remove to large plate.

4. Heat remaining ½ teaspoon oil in wok. Add mushrooms and snow peas; stir-fry 3 minutes or until snow peas are crisp-tender. Stir broth mixture; add to wok. Stir-fry 2 minutes or until sauce boils and thickens.

5. Return seafood and any accumulated juices to wok; stir-fry until heated through. Serve with rice; sprinkle with green onions.

NUTRITIONAL INFORMATION

Calories **304**, Total Fat **3g**, Saturated Fat **1g**, Cholesterol **74mg**, Sodium **335mg**, Carbohydrates **42g**, Dietary Fiber **3g**, Protein **25g**

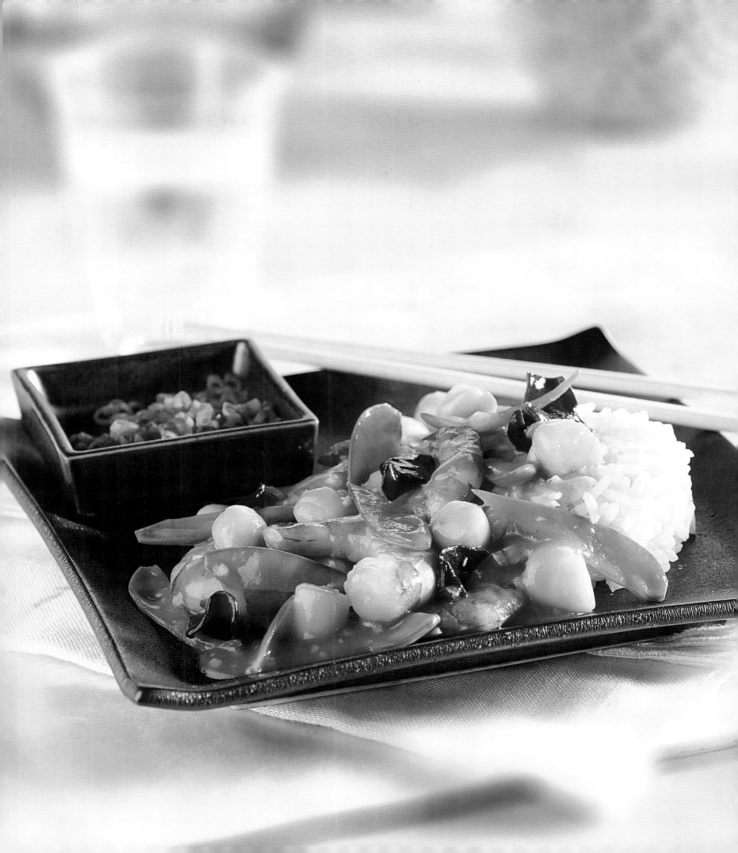

KALE & MUSHROOM STUFFED CHICKEN BREASTS

Makes 4 servings

3 teaspoons olive oil, divided

1 cup coarsely chopped mushrooms

2 cups thinly sliced kale

1 tablespoon fresh lemon juice

½ teaspoon salt, divided

4 boneless skinless chicken breasts (about 4 ounces each)

¼ cup crumbled fat-free feta cheese

¼ teaspoon black pepper

1. Heat 1 teaspoon oil in large skillet over medium-high heat. Add mushrooms; cook and stir 5 minutes or until mushrooms begin to brown. Add kale; cook and stir 8 minutes or until wilted. Sprinkle with lemon juice and ¼ teaspoon salt. Remove to small bowl. Let stand 5 to 10 minutes to cool slightly.

2. Meanwhile, place each chicken breast between sheets of plastic wrap. Pound with meat mallet or rolling pin to about ½-inch thickness.

3. Gently stir feta cheese into mushroom and kale mixture. Spoon ¼ cup mixture down center of each chicken breast. Roll up to enclose filling; secure with toothpicks. Sprinkle with remaining ¼ teaspoon salt and pepper.

4. Wipe out same skillet with paper towels. Add remaining 2 teaspoons oil to skillet; heat over medium heat. Add chicken; brown on all sides. Cover and cook 5 minutes per side or until no longer pink. Remove toothpicks before serving.

SERVING SUGGESTION: Serve this flavorful entrée with a fresh salad or summer vegetables.

NUTRITIONAL INFORMATION

Calories **192**, Total Fat **7g**, Saturated Fat **1g**, Cholesterol **73mg**, Sodium **495mg**, Carbohydrates **4g**, Dietary Fiber **1g**, Protein **29g**

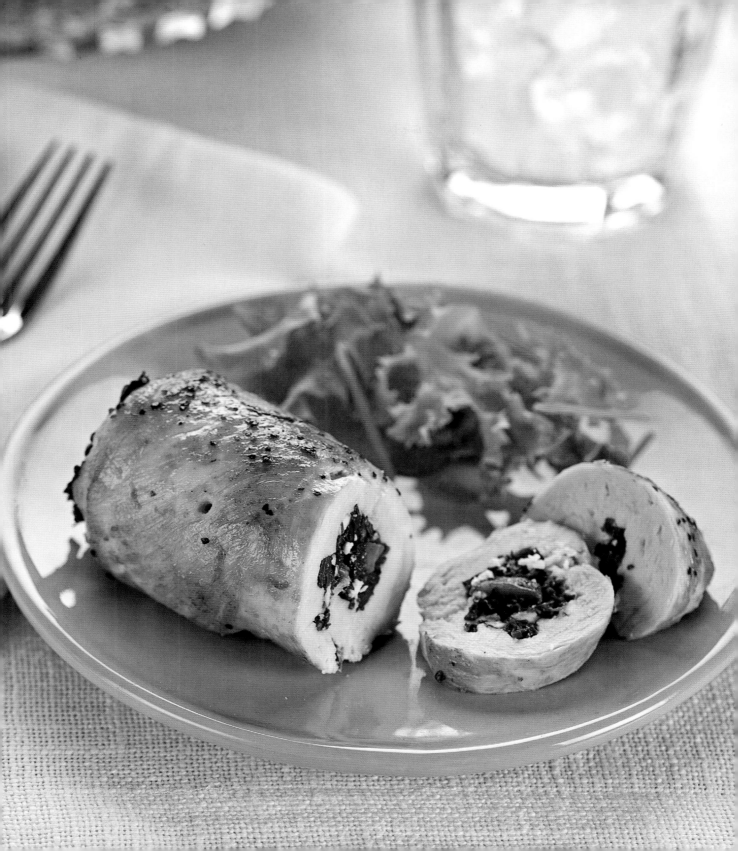

PASTA WITH SPINACH AND RICOTTA

Makes 4 servings

8 ounces uncooked tri-colored rotini pasta

1 package (10 ounces) frozen chopped spinach, thawed and squeezed dry

2 teaspoons minced garlic

1 cup fat-free or part-skim ricotta cheese

½ cup water

3 tablespoons grated Parmesan cheese, divided

Salt and black pepper

1. Cook pasta according to package directions. Drain well; cover and keep warm.

2. Spray large skillet with nonstick cooking spray; heat over medium-low heat. Add spinach and garlic; cook and stir 5 minutes. Stir in ricotta, water and 1½ tablespoons Parmesan cheese. Season with salt and pepper.

3. Add pasta to skillet; stir until well blended. Sprinkle with remaining 1½ tablespoons Parmesan cheese.

TIP: For a special touch, garnish with fresh basil leaves.

NUTRITIONAL INFORMATION

Calories **286**, Total Fat **2g**, Saturated Fat **1g**, Cholesterol **18mg**, Sodium **278mg**, Carbohydrates **48g**, Dietary Fiber **4g**, Protein **17g**

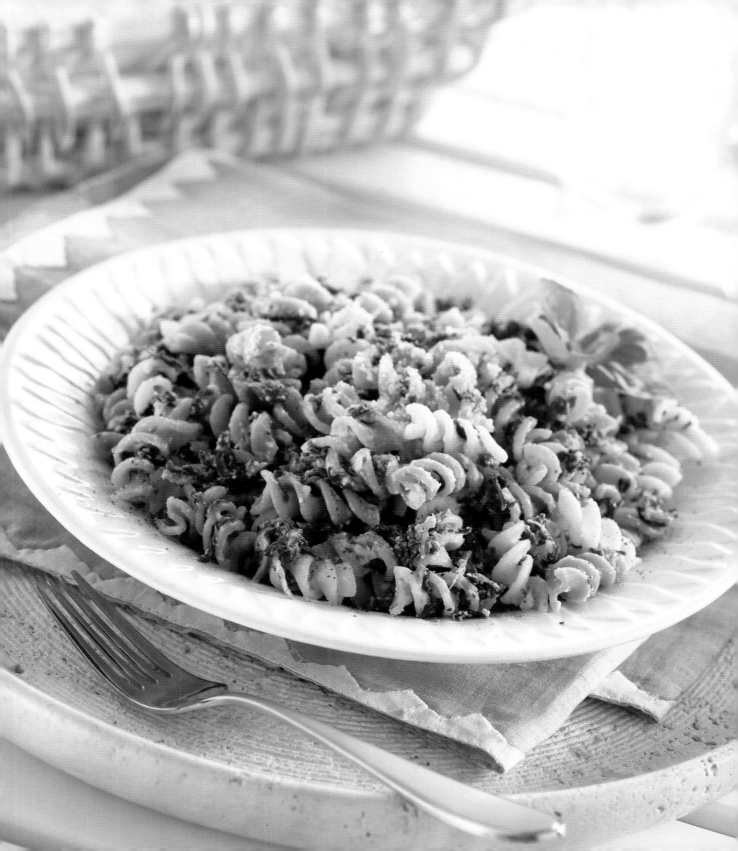

CRANBERRY CHUTNEY GLAZED SALMON

Makes 4 servings

½ teaspoon salt (optional)

½ teaspoon ground cinnamon

¼ teaspoon ground red pepper

4 skinless salmon fillets (5 to 6 ounces each)

¼ cup cranberry chutney

1 tablespoon white wine vinegar or cider vinegar

1. Preheat broiler or prepare grill for indirect cooking. Combine salt, if desired, cinnamon and red pepper in small bowl; rub over salmon. Combine chutney and vinegar in small bowl; brush about 1 tablespoon evenly over each salmon fillet.

2. Preheat broiler. Spray rack of broiler with nonstick cooking spray. Broil salmon 5 to 6 inches from heat source or grill over medium-hot coals on covered grill 4 to 6 minutes or until opaque in center.

VARIATION: If cranberry chutney is not available, substitute mango chutney. Chop any large pieces of mango.

NUTRITIONAL INFORMATION

Calories **229**, Total Fat **9g**, Saturated Fat **1g**, Cholesterol **78mg**, Sodium **104mg**, Carbohydrates **7g**, Dietary Fiber **1g**, Protein **28g**

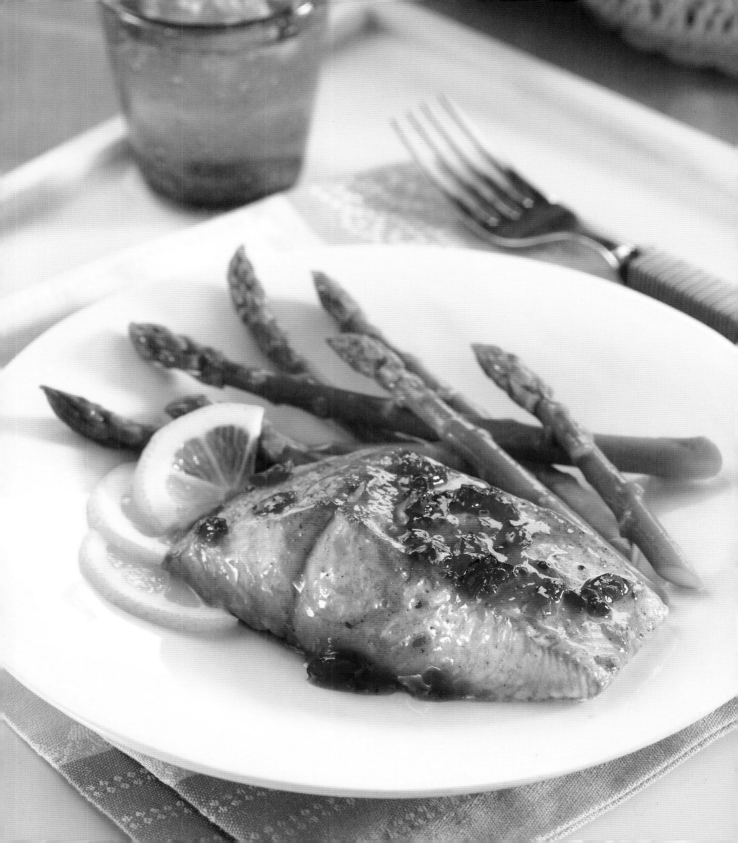

EASY MOO SHU PORK

Makes 2 servings

7 ounces pork tenderloin, sliced

4 green onions, cut into ½-inch pieces

1½ cups packaged coleslaw mix

2 tablespoons hoisin sauce or Asian plum sauce

4 (8-inch) fat-free flour tortillas, warmed

1. Spray large nonstick skillet with nonstick cooking spray; heat over medium-high heat. Add pork and green onions; stir-fry 2 to 3 minutes or until pork is barely pink. Stir in coleslaw mix and hoisin sauce.

2. Spoon pork mixture onto tortillas. Roll up tortillas, folding in sides to enclose filling.

NOTE: To warm tortillas, stack and wrap loosely in plastic wrap. Microwave on HIGH for 15 to 20 seconds or until hot and pliable.

NUTRITIONAL INFORMATION

Calories **293**, Total Fat **4g**, Saturated Fat **1g**, Cholesterol **58mg**, Sodium **672mg**, Carbohydrates **37g**, Dietary Fiber **14g**, Protein **26g**

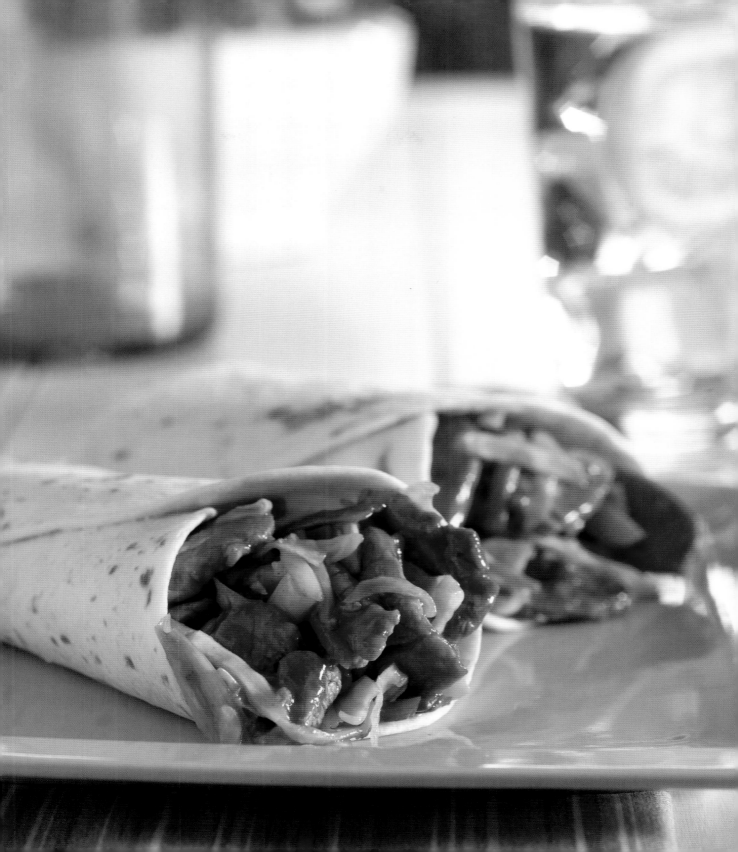

CHICKEN AND VEGGIE FAJITAS

Makes 6 servings

1 pound boneless skinless chicken thighs, cut crosswise into strips

1 teaspoon dried oregano

1 teaspoon chili powder

½ teaspoon garlic salt

2 bell peppers (preferably 1 red and 1 green), cut into thin strips

4 thin slices large sweet or yellow onion, separated into rings

½ cup salsa

6 (6-inch) flour tortillas, warmed

½ cup chopped fresh cilantro or green onions

Reduced-fat sour cream (optional)

1. Toss chicken with oregano, chili powder and garlic salt in large bowl. Heat large skillet coated with nonstick cooking spray over medium-high heat. Add chicken; cook and stir 5 to 6 minutes or until cooked through. Remove to bowl; set aside.

2. Add bell peppers and onion to same skillet; cook and stir 2 minutes over medium heat. Add salsa; cover and cook 6 to 8 minutes or until vegetables are tender. Uncover; stir in chicken and any juices from bowl. Cook and stir 2 minutes or until heated through.

3. Serve mixture on top of tortillas topped with cilantro and sour cream, if desired.

NUTRITIONAL INFORMATION

Calories **159**, Total Fat **5g**, Saturated Fat **1g**, Cholesterol **63mg**, Sodium **476mg**, Carbohydrates **15g**, Dietary Fiber **8g**, Protein **21g**

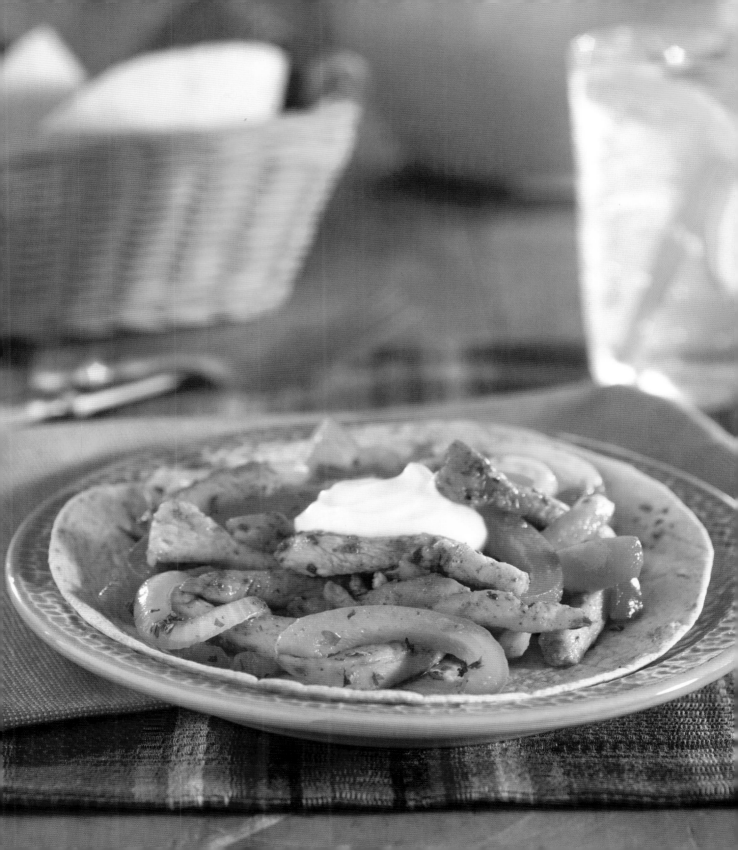

CHICKEN & WILD RICE SKILLET DINNER

Makes 1 serving

1 teaspoon reduced-fat margarine

2 ounces boneless skinless chicken breast, cut into strips (about ½ chicken breast)

1 package (5 ounces) long grain and wild rice mix with seasoning

½ cup water

3 dried apricots, cut up

1. Melt margarine in small skillet over medium-high heat. Add chicken; cook and stir 3 to 5 minutes or until cooked through.

2. Meanwhile, measure ¼ cup of the rice and 1 tablespoon plus ½ teaspoon of the seasoning mix. Reserve remaining rice and seasoning mix for another use.

3. Add rice, seasoning mix, water and apricots to skillet; mix well. Bring to a boil. Cover and reduce heat to low; simmer 25 minutes or until liquid is absorbed and rice is tender.

NUTRITIONAL INFORMATION

Calories **314**, Total Fat **5g**, Saturated Fat **1g**, Cholesterol **52mg**, Sodium **669mg**, Carbohydrates **44g**, Dietary Fiber **3g**, Protein **24g**

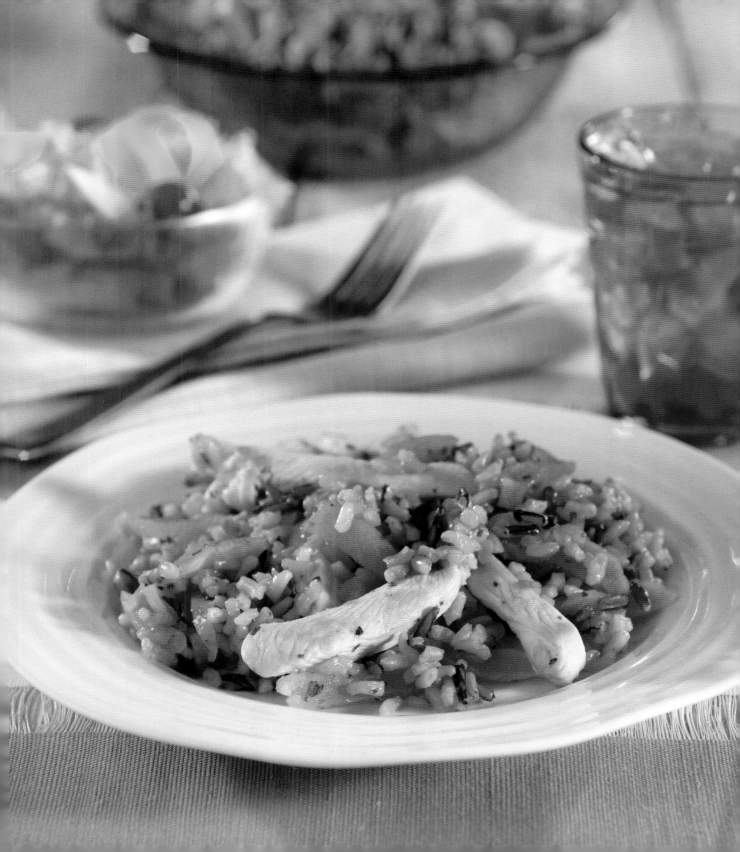

WHOLE WHEAT PENNE WITH BROCCOLI AND SAUSAGE

Makes 6 servings

6 to 7 ounces uncooked whole wheat penne pasta

8 ounces broccoli florets

8 ounces mild Italian turkey sausage, casings removed

1 medium onion, quartered and sliced

2 cloves garlic, minced

2 teaspoons grated lemon peel

¼ teaspoon salt

⅛ teaspoon black pepper

⅓ cup grated Parmesan cheese

1. Cook pasta according to package directions, omitting salt. Add broccoli during last 5 to 6 minutes of cooking. Drain well; cover and keep warm.

2. Meanwhile, heat large nonstick skillet over medium heat. Crumble sausage into skillet. Add onion; cook until sausage is brown, stirring to break up meat. Drain fat. Add garlic; cook and stir 1 minute.

3. Add sausage mixture, lemon peel, salt and pepper to pasta mixture; toss until blended. Sprinkle Parmesan cheese evenly over each serving.

NUTRITIONAL INFORMATION

Calories **208**, Total Fat **6g**, Saturated Fat **1g**, Cholesterol **26mg**, Sodium **425mg**, Carbohydrates **26g**, Dietary Fiber **4g**, Protein **13g**

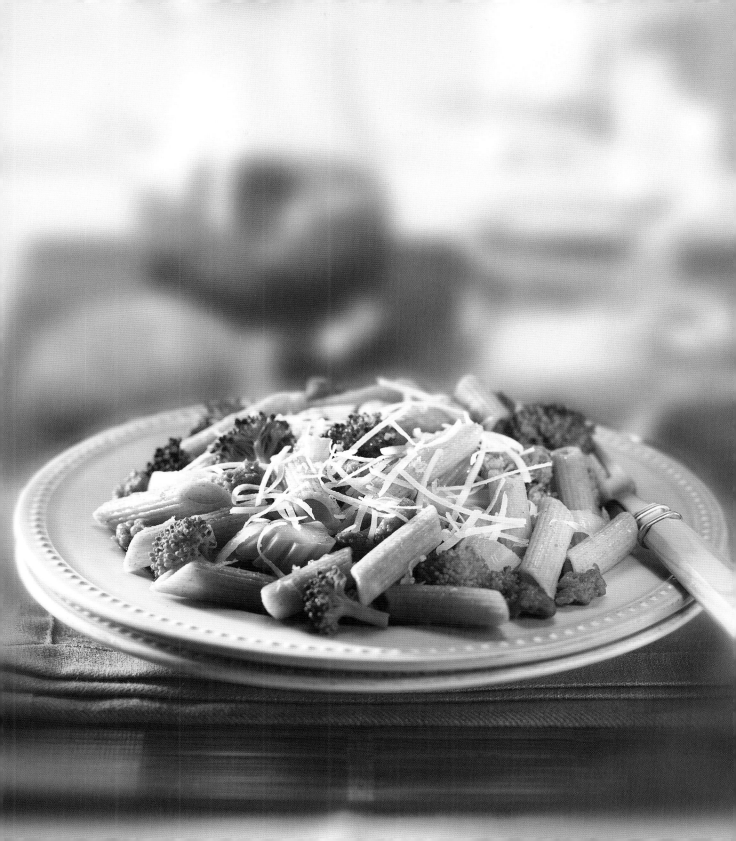

ROASTED ALMOND TILAPIA

Makes 2 servings

2 tilapia or Boston scrod fillets (6 ounces each)

¼ teaspoon salt

1 tablespoon prepared mustard

¼ cup whole wheat bread crumbs

2 tablespoons chopped almonds

Paprika (optional)

Lemon wedges (optional)

1. Preheat oven to 450°F. Place fish on small baking sheet; season with salt. Spread mustard over fish. Combine bread crumbs and almonds in small bowl; sprinkle over fish. Press lightly to adhere. Sprinkle with paprika, if desired.

2. Bake 8 to 10 minutes or until fish is opaque in center and begins to flake when tested with fork. Serve with lemon wedges, if desired.

NUTRITIONAL INFORMATION

Calories **240**, Total Fat **6g**, Saturated Fat **1g**, Cholesterol **85mg**, Sodium **470mg**, Carbohydrates **9g**, Dietary Fiber **1g**, Protein **37g**

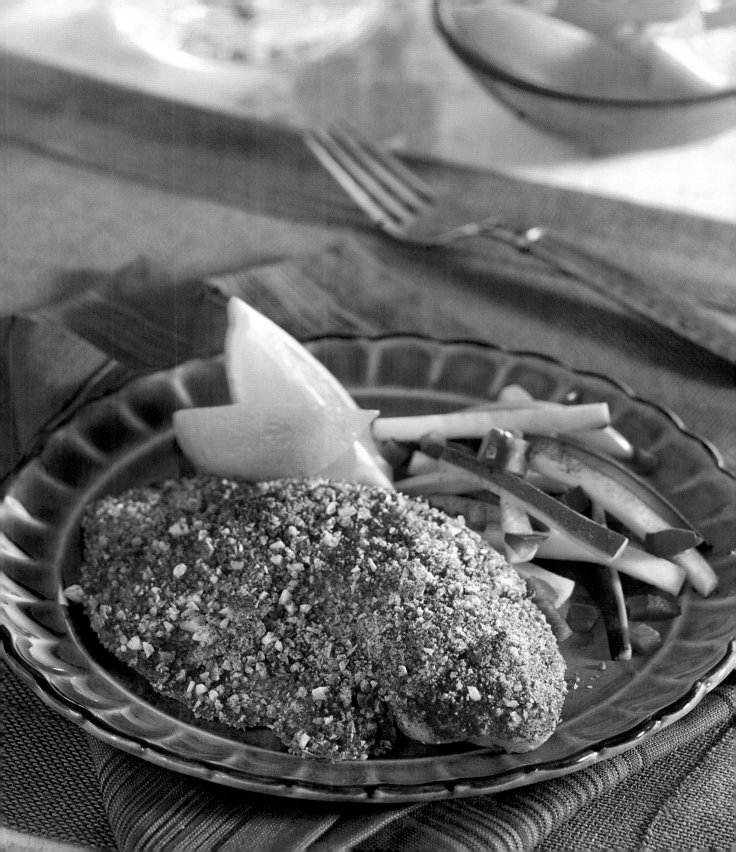

HAMBURGERS WITH ZUCCHINI AND RED ONION

Makes 4 servings

¾ pound extra-lean ground beef

⅓ cup shredded zucchini*

2 tablespoons minced red onion

½ teaspoon dried thyme

¼ teaspoon kosher salt (optional)

⅛ teaspoon black pepper

Wash the zucchini well before using a grater to shred it.

1. Combine beef, zucchini, onion, thyme, salt, if desired, and pepper in large bowl. Shape into four 3-inch patties.

2. Lightly coat large skillet with nonstick cooking spray; heat over medium heat. Add patties and cook 8 minutes, turning occasionally, or until cooked through.

SPAGHETTI BOLOGNESE: Save 2 hamburgers; cut into small chunks. Coat large skillet with nonstick cooking spray; heat over medium heat. Add burgers, 1 cup diced carrots and ⅓ cup diced celery; cook stirring occasionally, 6 to 7 minutes or until vegetables are softened. Add 1 can (about 14 ounces) no-salt-added diced tomatoes (undrained), ½ cup reduced-fat (2%) milk, 1 tablespoon tomato paste, ¼ teaspoon kosher salt, if desired, ⅛ teaspoon ground nutmeg and ⅛ teaspoon black pepper. Stir and bring to a boil; reduce heat and simmer, stirring occasionally, 6 to 8 minutes or until lightly thickened. Serve over hot cooked whole grain spaghetti.

NUTRITIONAL INFORMATION

Calories **112**, Total Fat **3.5g**, Saturated Fat **1.5g**, Cholesterol **45mg**, Sodium **56mg**, Carbohydrates **14g**, Dietary Fiber **1g**, Protein **18g**

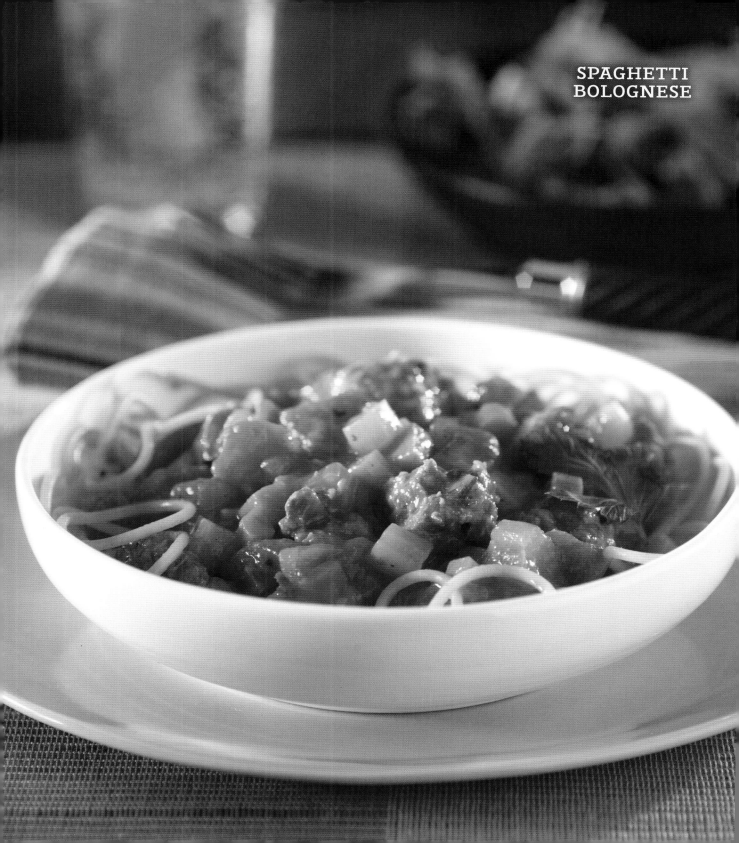

SPAGHETTI
BOLOGNESE

SKILLET FISH WITH LEMON TARRAGON "BUTTER"

Makes 2 servings

2 teaspoons reduced-fat margarine

4 teaspoons lemon juice, divided

½ teaspoon grated lemon peel

¼ teaspoon prepared mustard

¼ teaspoon dried tarragon

⅛ teaspoon salt

2 lean white fish fillets (4 ounces each),* rinsed and patted dry

¼ teaspoon paprika

Cod, orange roughy, flounder, haddock, halibut and sole can be used.

1. Combine margarine, 2 teaspoons lemon juice, lemon peel, mustard, tarragon and salt in small bowl; mix well with fork.

2. Spray 12-inch nonstick skillet with nonstick cooking spray; heat over medium heat. Drizzle fish with remaining 2 teaspoons lemon juice; sprinkle one side of each fillet with paprika.

3. Place fish in skillet, paprika side down; cook 3 minutes. Gently turn and cook 3 minutes longer or until fish is opaque in center and begins to flake when tested with fork. Top with margarine mixture.

NUTRITIONAL INFORMATION

Calories **125**, Total Fat **3g**, Saturated Fat **1g**, Cholesterol **60mg**, Sodium **291mg**, Carbohydrates **1g**, Dietary Fiber **1g**, Protein **22g**

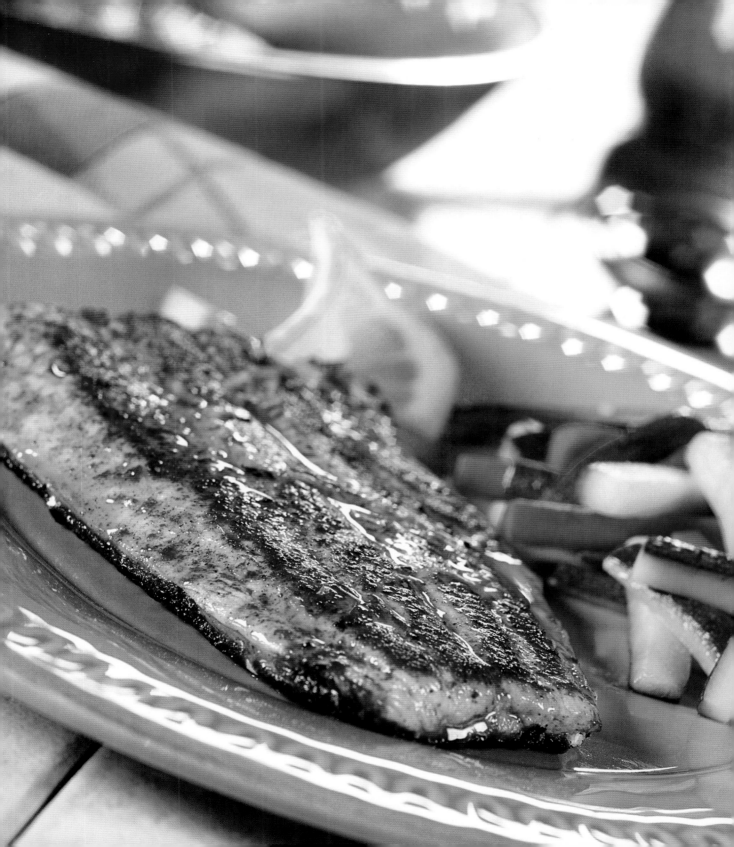

GRILLED PORK FAJITAS WITH MANGO AND SALSA VERDE

Makes 4 servings (2 fajitas per serving)

2 cloves garlic, crushed

2 teaspoons chili powder

½ teaspoon ground cumin

½ teaspoon ground coriander

12 ounces pork tenderloin, trimmed of fat

1 medium red onion, cut into ½-inch rings

1 mango, peeled and cut into ½-inch pieces

8 (6-inch) flour tortillas, warmed

½ cup salsa verde

1. Spray grid with nonstick cooking spray. Prepare grill for direct cooking over medium-high heat.

2. Combine garlic, chili powder, cumin and coriander in small bowl. Rub evenly onto pork.

3. Grill pork 12 to 16 minutes or until thermometer registers 155°F for medium doneness, turning occasionally. During last 8 minutes of grilling, grill onion until tender, turning occasionally.

4. Remove onion to small bowl. Remove pork to cutting board; tent loosely with foil. Let stand 5 to 10 minutes before slicing into ½-inch strips.

5. Arrange pork, onion and mango on tortillas. Spoon evenly with salsa verde. Fold bottom 3 inches of each tortilla up over filling; roll up to enclose filling.

NUTRITIONAL INFORMATION

Calories **270**, Total Fat **2g**, Saturated Fat **1g**, Cholesterol **55mg**, Sodium **713mg**, Carbohydrates **38g**, Dietary Fiber **6g**, Protein **25g**

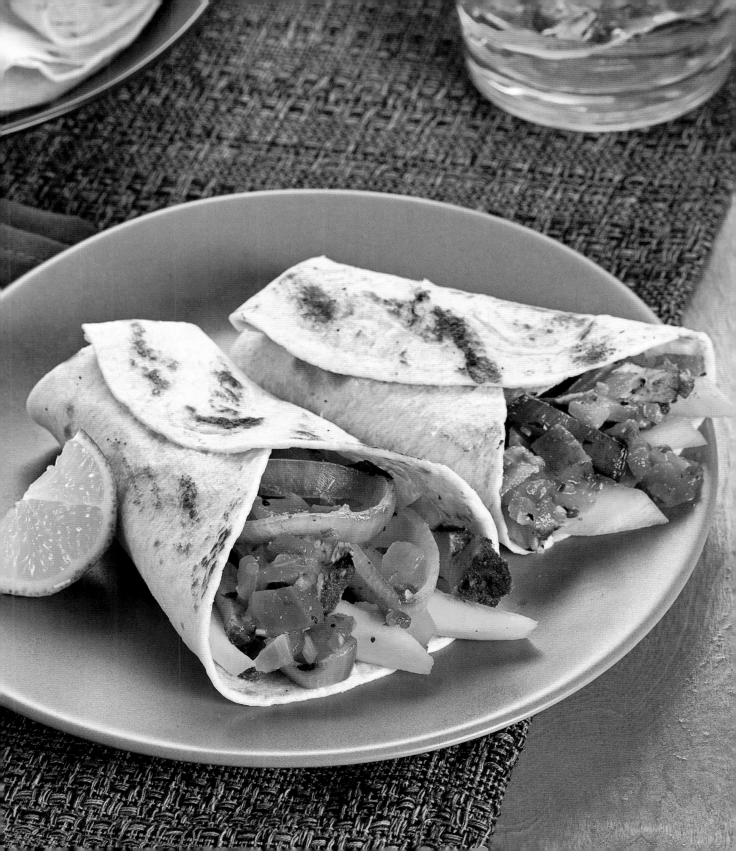

CHICKEN PICCATA

Makes 4 servings

3 tablespoons all-purpose flour

½ teaspoon salt

¼ teaspoon black pepper

4 boneless skinless chicken breasts
   (4 ounces each)

2 teaspoons olive oil

1 teaspoon butter

2 cloves garlic, minced

¾ cup fat-free reduced-sodium
   chicken broth

1 tablespoon fresh lemon juice

2 tablespoons chopped fresh
   Italian parsley

1 tablespoon capers, drained

1. Combine flour, salt and pepper in shallow dish. Reserve 1 tablespoon flour mixture.

2. Pound chicken between waxed paper to ½-inch thickness with flat side of meat mallet or rolling pin. Coat chicken with flour mixture, shaking off excess.

3. Heat oil and butter in large nonstick skillet over medium heat. Add chicken; cook 4 to 5 minutes per side or until no longer pink in center. Transfer to serving platter; cover loosely with foil.

4. Add garlic to same skillet; cook and stir 1 minute. Add reserved flour mixture; cook and stir 1 minute. Add broth and lemon juice; cook 2 minutes or until thickened, stirring frequently. Stir in parsley and capers; spoon sauce over chicken.

NUTRITIONAL INFORMATION

Calories **194**, Total Fat **6g**, Saturated Fat **2g**, Cholesterol **71mg**,
Sodium **473mg**, Carbohydrates **5g**, Dietary Fiber **1g**, Protein **27g**

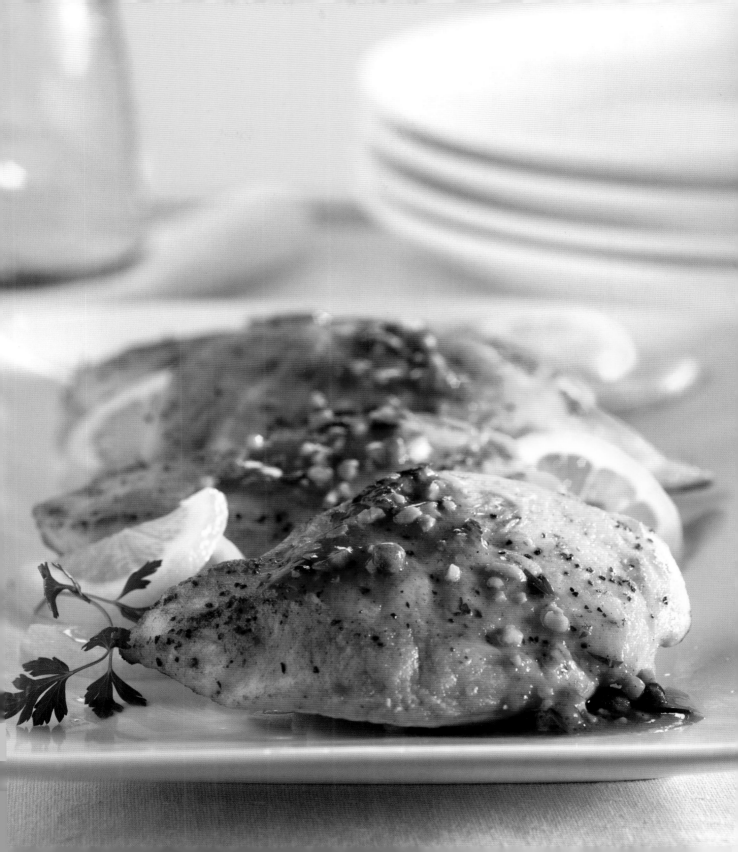

MAPLE & SAGE PORK CHOPS

Makes 4 servings

2 tablespoons finely chopped fresh sage, plus additional for garnish

2 teaspoons olive oil

½ teaspoon salt

4 boneless pork chops (about 4 ounces each)

2 teaspoons maple syrup

1. Combine 2 tablespoons sage, oil and salt in small bowl. Rub mixture evenly over pork chops. Place on rimmed baking sheet.

2. Preheat broiler. Broil pork chops 4 minutes. Turn over; brush evenly with maple syrup. Broil 4 minutes or until pork chops are browned and barely pink in center. Garnish with additional sage.

SERVING SUGGESTION: This delicious dish is perfect for a cold day. Serve it with fresh roasted vegetables to combine the unique flavors of fall with the delightful flavor of the tender pork.

NUTRITIONAL INFORMATION

Calories **203**, Total Fat **10g**, Saturated Fat **3g**, Cholesterol **62mg**, Sodium **342mg**, Carbohydrates **2g**, Dietary Fiber **1g**, Protein **25g**

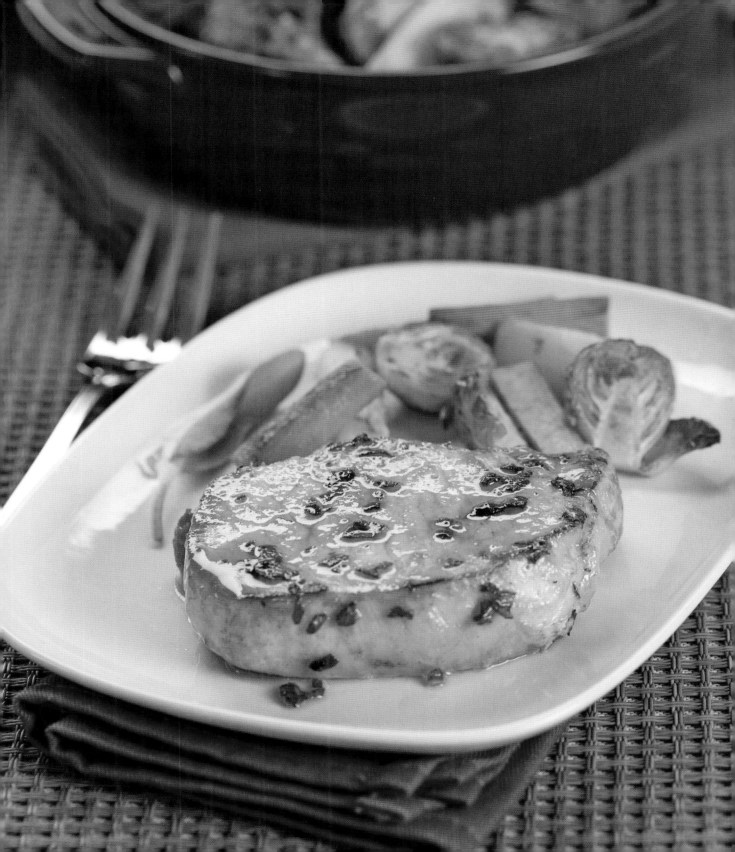

PENNE PASTA WITH CHUNKY TOMATO SAUCE AND SPINACH

Makes 8 servings

8 ounces uncooked multigrain penne pasta

2 cups spicy marinara sauce

1 large ripe tomato, chopped (about 1½ cups)

4 cups packed baby spinach or torn spinach leaves (4 ounces)

¼ cup grated Parmesan cheese

¼ cup chopped fresh basil

1. Cook pasta according to package directions, omitting salt.

2. Meanwhile, heat marinara sauce and tomato in medium saucepan over medium heat 3 to 4 minutes or until hot and bubbly, stirring occasionally. Remove from heat; stir in spinach.

3. Drain pasta; return to saucepan. Add sauce; toss to combine. Divide evenly among eight serving bowls; top with cheese and basil.

NUTRITIONAL INFORMATION

Calories **171**, Total Fat **3g**, Saturated Fat **1g**, Cholesterol **4mg**, Sodium **319mg**, Carbohydrates **29g**, Dietary Fiber **4g**, Protein **7g**

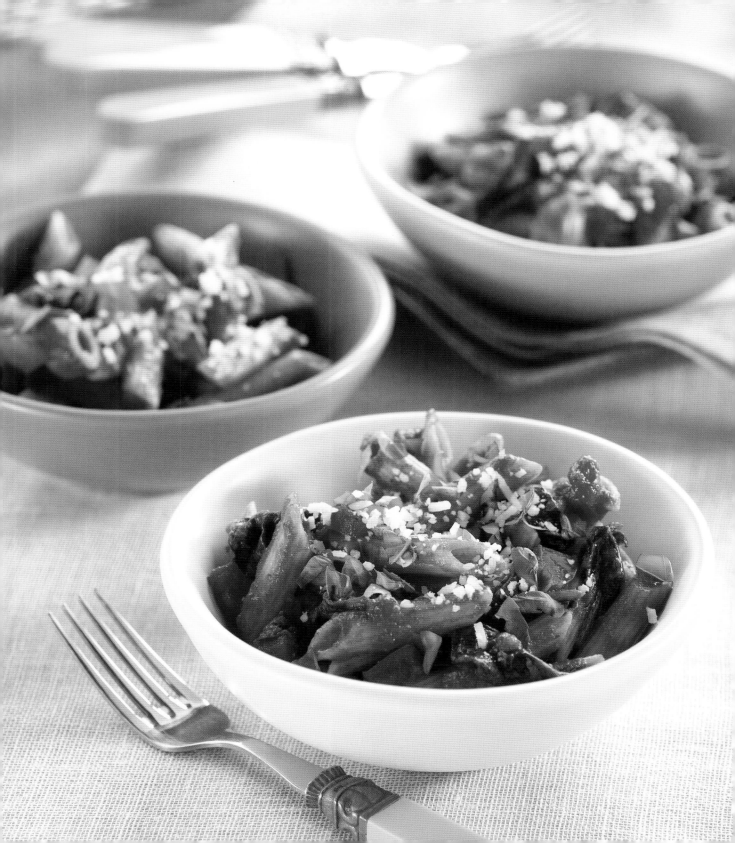

ROAST DILL SCROD
WITH ASPARAGUS

Makes 4 servings

1 bunch (12 ounces) asparagus spears, ends trimmed

1 teaspoon olive oil

4 scrod or cod fillets (about 5 ounces each)

1 tablespoon lemon juice

1 teaspoon dried dill weed

½ teaspoon salt

¼ teaspoon black pepper

Paprika (optional)

1. Preheat oven to 425°F.

2. Place asparagus in 13×9-inch baking dish; drizzle with oil. Roll asparagus to coat lightly with oil; push to edges of dish, stacking asparagus into two layers.

3. Arrange fish fillets in center of dish; drizzle with lemon juice. Combine dill weed, salt and pepper in small bowl; sprinkle over fish and asparagus. Sprinkle with paprika, if desired.

4. Roast 15 to 17 minutes or until asparagus is crisp-tender and fish is opaque in center and begins to flake when tested with fork.

NUTRITIONAL INFORMATION

Calories **147**, Total Fat **2g**, Saturated Fat **1g**, Cholesterol **61mg**, Sodium **379mg**, Carbohydrates **4g**, Dietary Fiber **2g**, Protein **27g**

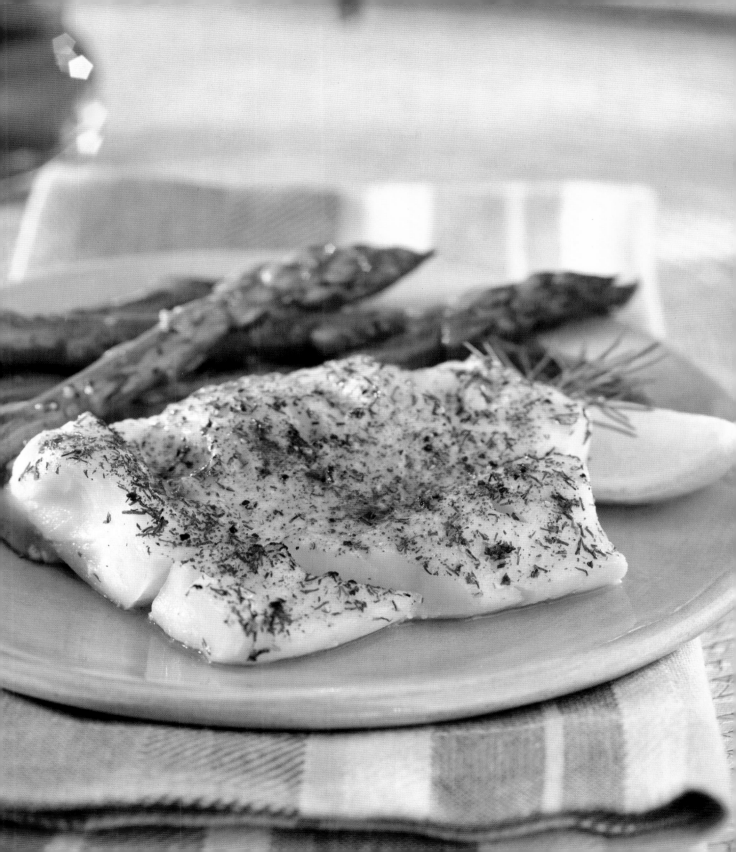

GROUND BEEF, SPINACH AND BARLEY SOUP

Makes 4 servings

¾ pound lean ground beef

4 cups water

1 can (about 14 ounces) stewed tomatoes

1½ cups thinly sliced carrots

1 cup chopped onion

½ cup uncooked quick-cooking barley

1½ teaspoons beef bouillon granules

1½ teaspoons dried thyme

1 teaspoon dried oregano

½ teaspoon garlic powder

¼ teaspoon black pepper

⅛ teaspoon salt

3 cups fresh spinach leaves

1. Brown beef in large saucepan over medium-high heat 6 to 8 minutes, stirring to break up meat. Rinse beef under warm water; drain.

2. Return beef to saucepan; stir in water, tomatoes, carrots, onion, barley, bouillon granules, thyme, oregano, garlic powder, pepper and salt; bring to a boil over high heat.

3. Reduce heat to medium-low. Cover; simmer 12 to 15 minutes or until barley and vegetables are tender, stirring occasionally. Stir in spinach; cook until spinach starts to wilt.

NUTRITIONAL INFORMATION

Calories **265**, Total Fat **6g**, Saturated Fat **2g**, Cholesterol **22mg**, Sodium **512mg**, Carbohydrates **33g**, Dietary Fiber **8g**, Protein **22g**

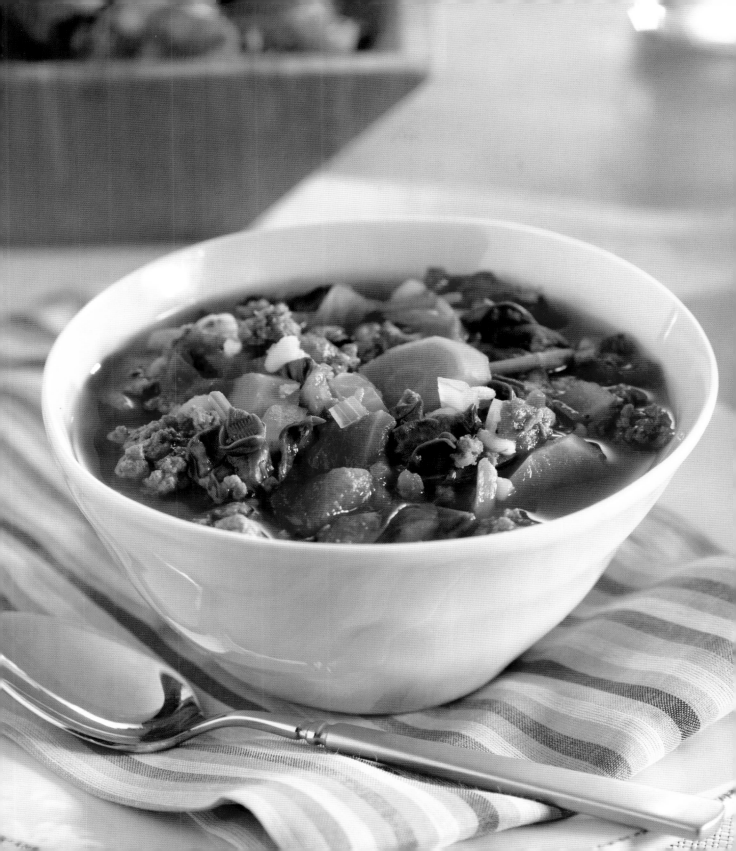

BROILED SALMON WITH CUCUMBER YOGURT

Makes 4 servings

1 cup plain nonfat yogurt

⅔ cup finely chopped cucumber

1 pound salmon fillet, cut into 4 pieces

2 teaspoons honey

1 teaspoon Dijon mustard

¼ teaspoon curry powder

1. Combine yogurt and cucumber in medium bowl; cover and refrigerate.

2. Preheat broiler. Place salmon, skin side down, on foil-lined baking sheet. Stir honey, mustard and curry powder in small bowl until smooth. Spread on salmon. Broil about 5 inches from heat 10 minutes or until opaque in center. Serve with cucumber yogurt.

SERVING SUGGESTION: Serve with brown rice pilaf and asparagus. Be sure to prepare your side dishes without excess oil, butter or salt.

NUTRITIONAL INFORMATION

Calories **252**, Total Fat **12g**, Saturated Fat **3g**, Cholesterol **57mg**, Sodium **111mg**, Carbohydrates **9g**, Dietary Fiber **0g**, Protein **26g**

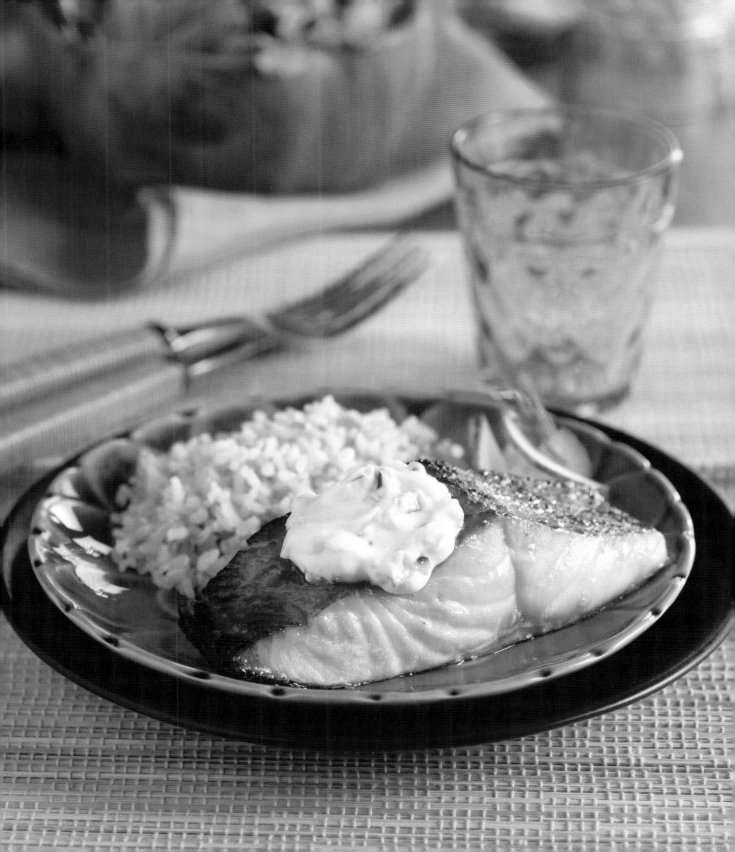

THAI GRILLED CHICKEN

Makes 4 servings

4 boneless skinless chicken breasts (about 1¼ pounds)

¼ cup low-sodium soy sauce

2 teaspoons minced garlic

½ teaspoon red pepper flakes

2 tablespoons honey

1 tablespoon fresh lime juice

1. Prepare grill for direct cooking over medium heat. Place chicken in shallow baking dish. Combine soy sauce, garlic and red pepper flakes in small bowl. Pour over chicken, turning to coat. Let stand 10 minutes.

2. Meanwhile, combine honey and lime juice in small bowl; blend well. Set aside.

3. Place chicken on grid; brush with marinade. Discard remaining marinade. Grill, covered, 5 minutes. Brush both sides of chicken with honey mixture. Grill 5 minutes more or until chicken is no longer pink in center.

SERVING SUGGESTION: Serve with steamed white rice, Oriental vegetables and a fresh fruit salad.

NUTRITIONAL INFORMATION

Calories **140**, Total Fat **1g**, Saturated Fat **1g**, Cholesterol **53mg**, Sodium **349mg**, Carbohydrates **10g**, Dietary Fiber **1g**, Protein **22g**

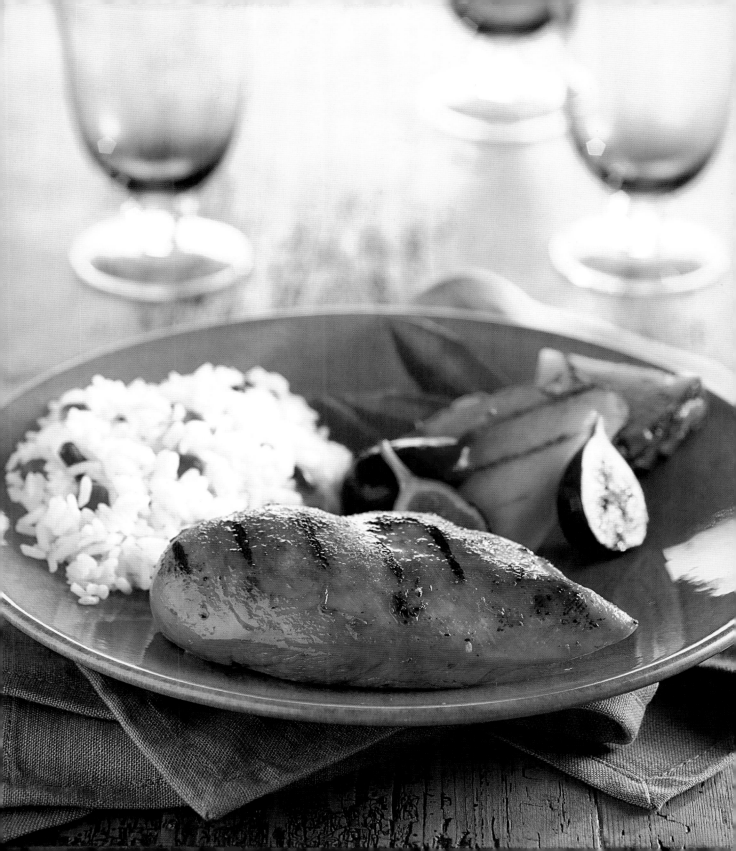

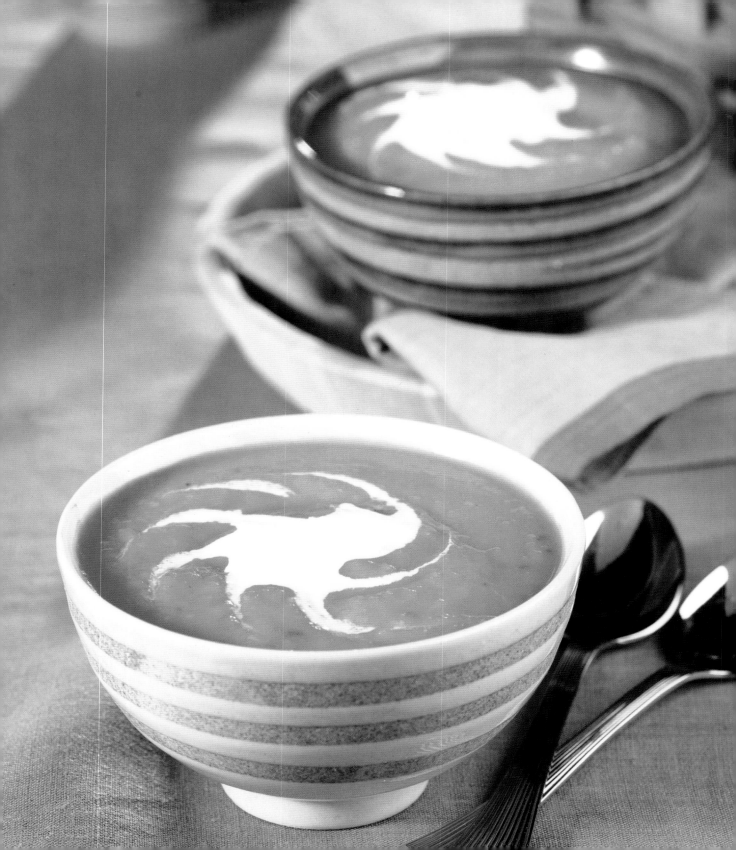

SOUPS & SIDES

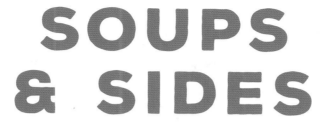

WINTER SQUASH SOUP

Makes 4 servings

1 tablespoon reduced-fat margarine

1 tablespoon minced shallot or onion

2 cloves garlic, minced

3 fresh thyme sprigs

Pinch dried rosemary

2 packages (10 ounces each) frozen butternut squash, thawed

1 cup fat-free reduced-sodium chicken broth

3 tablespoons fat-free (skim) milk

Fat-free sour cream (optional)

1. Melt margarine in medium saucepan over medium heat. Add shallot, garlic, thyme and rosemary; cook and stir 2 to 3 minutes or until shallot is tender. Add squash and broth; bring to a boil. Add milk; stir until blended.

2. Remove and discard thyme. Working in batches, process soup in blender or food processor until smooth. (Add additional broth or water to make soup thinner, if desired.) Top each serving with dollop of sour cream, if desired.

NUTRITIONAL INFORMATION

Calories **116**, Total Fat **2g**, Saturated Fat **1g**, Cholesterol **1mg**, Sodium **135mg**, Carbohydrates **22g**, Dietary Fiber **2g**, Protein **5g**

QUICK ZUCCHINI PARMESAN

Makes 4 servings

2 teaspoons olive oil

2 large zucchini or yellow squash, cut into ¼-inch thick slices (4 cups)

2 cloves garlic, minced

¼ teaspoon black pepper

¼ teaspoon salt (optional)

¼ cup thinly sliced basil

2 tablespoons grated Parmesan cheese

Heat oil in large nonstick skillet over medium heat. Add zucchini; cook and stir 2 minutes. Add garlic, pepper and salt, if desired; cook 4 to 5 minutes or just until zucchini is tender. Top with basil and cheese.

NUTRITIONAL INFORMATION

Calories **50**, Total Fat **3g**, Saturated Fat **1g**, Cholesterol **2mg**, Sodium **48mg**, Carbohydrates **4g**, Dietary Fiber **1g**, Protein **2g**

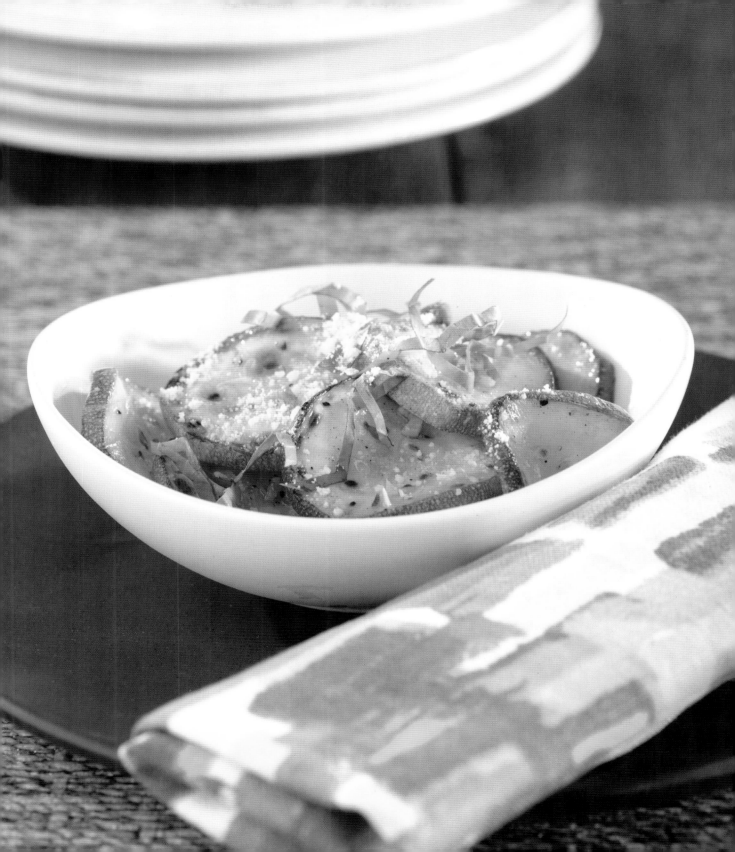

MANDARIN CHICKEN SALAD

Makes 4 servings

3½ ounces thin rice noodles (rice vermicelli)

1 can (6 ounces) mandarin orange segments, chilled

⅓ cup honey

2 tablespoons rice wine vinegar

2 tablespoons reduced-sodium soy sauce

1 can (8 ounces) sliced water chestnuts, drained

4 cups shredded napa cabbage

1 cup shredded red cabbage

½ cup sliced radishes

4 thin slices red onion, cut in half and separated

3 boneless skinless chicken breasts (about 12 ounces), cooked and cut into strips

1. Place rice noodles in large bowl. Cover with hot water; soak 20 minutes or until soft. Drain.

2. Drain mandarin orange segments, reserving ⅓ cup liquid. Whisk reserved liquid, honey, vinegar and soy sauce in medium bowl. Add water chestnuts.

3. Divide noodles, cabbages, radishes and onion evenly among four serving plates. Top with chicken and orange segments. Remove water chestnuts from dressing and arrange on salads. Serve with remaining dressing.

NUTRITIONAL INFORMATION

Calories **258**, Total Fat **2g**, Saturated Fat **1g**, Cholesterol **34mg**, Sodium **318mg**, Carbohydrates **46g**, Dietary Fiber **2g**, Protein **16g**

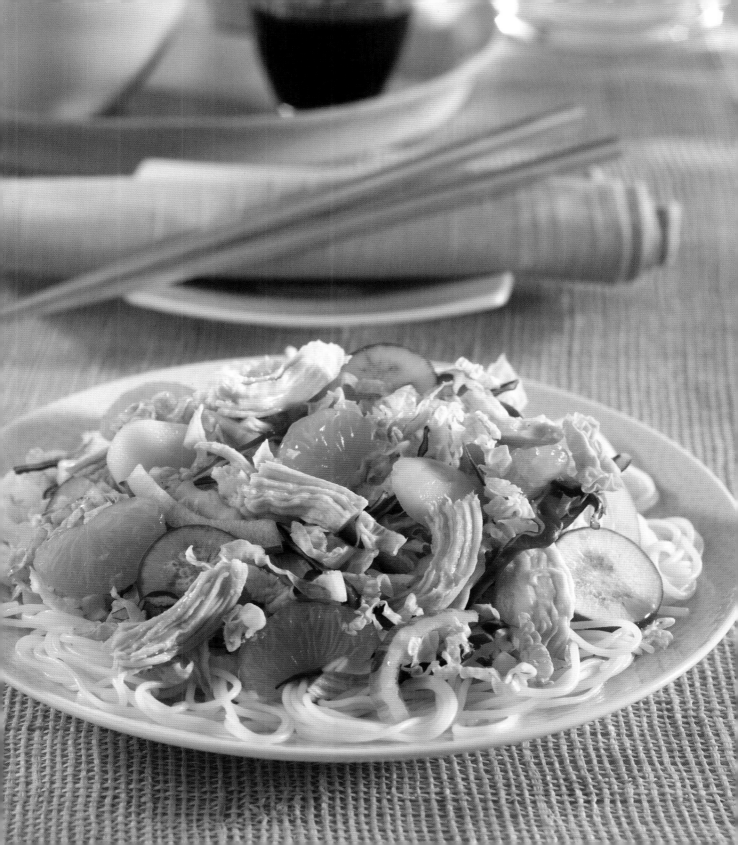

TOMATO-HERB SOUP

Makes 4 servings

1 can (about 14 ounces) no-salt-added diced tomatoes

1 can (about 14 ounces) reduced-sodium chicken broth

1 package (8 ounces) frozen bell pepper stir-fry mixture

1 cup frozen green beans

½ cup water

1 tablespoon ketchup

1 to 2 teaspoons dried oregano

1 teaspoon dried basil

⅛ teaspoon red pepper flakes (optional)

Combine tomatoes, broth, bell peppers, green beans, water, ketchup, oregano, basil and red pepper flakes, if desired, in large saucepan. Bring to a boil over medium-high heat. Reduce heat to medium-low. Simmer, covered, 20 minutes or until beans are tender.

VARIATION: Substitute chopped fresh bell peppers for the frozen stir-fry mix.

NUTRITIONAL INFORMATION

Calories **94**, Total Fat **3g**, Saturated Fat **1g**, Cholesterol **0mg**, Sodium **327mg**, Carbohydrates **14g**, Dietary Fiber **4g**, Protein **3g**

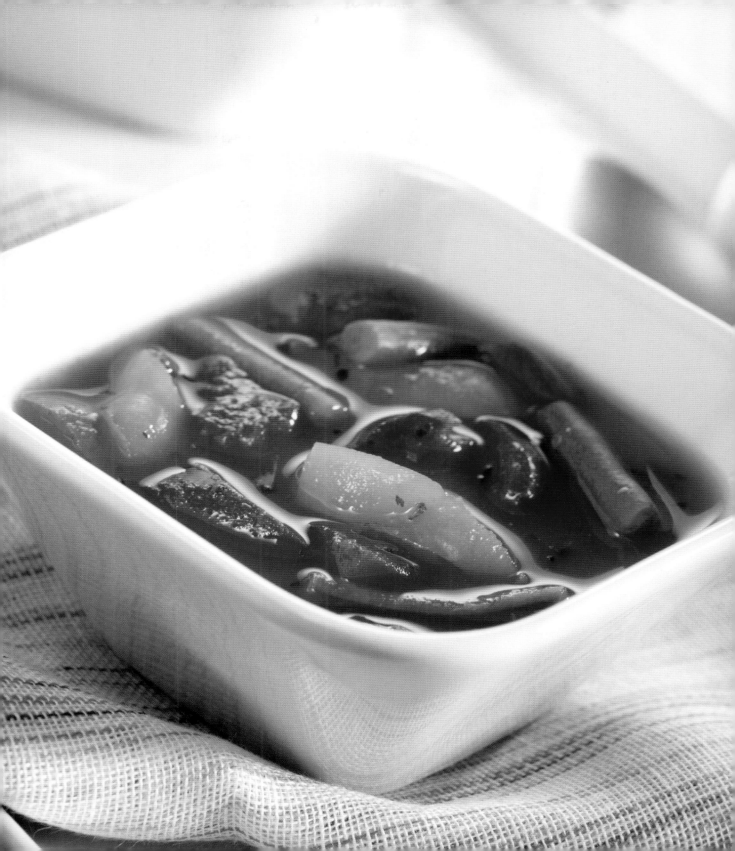

SANTA FE ROTINI

Makes 2 servings

3 ounces uncooked whole grain rotini pasta

½ of 15-ounce can black beans, rinsed and drained

⅓ cup finely chopped red onion

1 medium jalapeño pepper,* seeded and chopped

¾ cup quartered grape tomatoes

1 tablespoon extra virgin olive oil

½ lime, cut into 4 wedges, divided

1 clove garlic, minced

⅛ teaspoon salt

1 to 2 tablespoons chopped fresh cilantro (optional)

Jalapeño peppers can sting and irritate the skin, so wear rubber gloves when handling peppers and do not touch your eyes.

1. Cook pasta according to package directions omitting any salt or fat. Add beans during last minute of cooking. Drain.

2. Meanwhile, coat small nonstick skillet with nonstick cooking spray; heat over medium-high heat. Add onion and jalapeño pepper; cook 2 minutes, stirring frequently. Add tomatoes; cook 2 minutes or until just tender, stirring frequently. Remove from heat; cover and set aside.

3. In small bowl, combine oil, juice of 2 lime wedges, garlic and salt.

4. Place pasta mixture on two dinner plates. Stir oil mixture into tomato mixture until just coated; spoon evenly over pasta. Sprinkle evenly with cilantro, if desired. Serve with remaining lime wedges.

TIP: Freeze remaining beans in an airtight container for later use for up to 1 month.

NUTRITIONAL INFORMATION

Calories **298**, Total Fat **8g**, Saturated Fat **1g**, Cholesterol **0mg**, Sodium **571mg**, Carbohydrates **50g**, Dietary Fiber **10g**, Protein **13g**

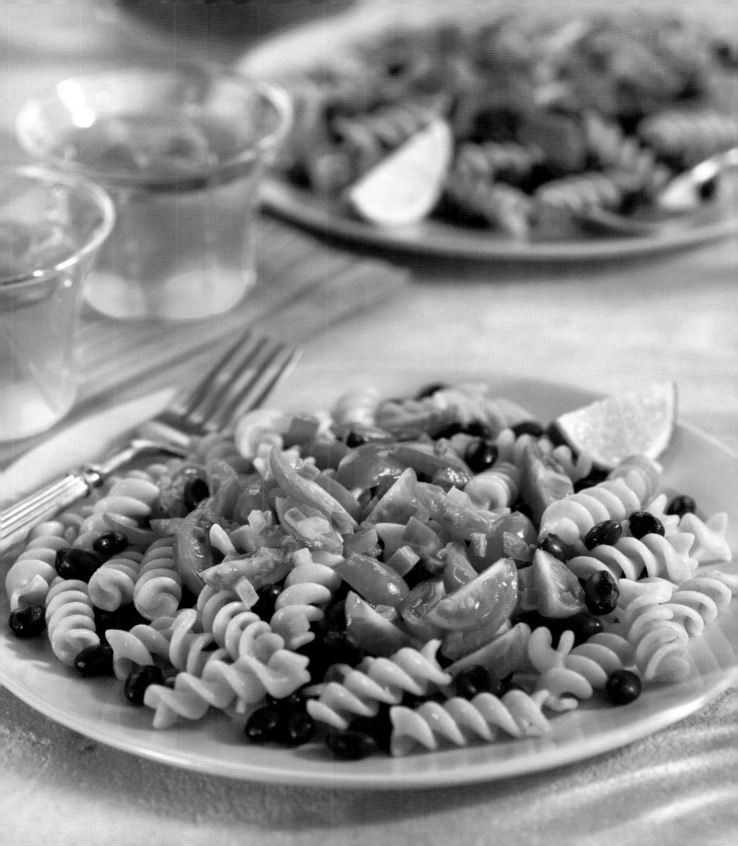

MASHED POTATO PUFFS

Makes 18 puffs (3 puffs per serving)

1 cup prepared mashed potatoes

½ cup finely chopped broccoli *or* spinach

2 egg whites

4 tablespoons shredded Parmesan cheese, divided

1. Preheat oven to 400°F. Spray 18 mini (1¾-inch) muffin cups with nonstick cooking spray.

2. Combine mashed potatoes, broccoli, egg whites and 2 tablespoons cheese in large bowl; mix well. Spoon evenly into prepared muffin cups. Sprinkle with remaining 2 tablespoons cheese.

3. Bake 20 to 23 minutes or until golden brown. To remove from pan, gently run knife around outer edges and lift out with fork. Serve warm.

NUTRITIONAL INFORMATION

Calories **63**, Total Fat **2g**, Saturated Fat **1g**, Cholesterol **2mg**, Sodium **99mg**, Carbohydrates **8g**, Dietary Fiber **1g**, Protein **32g**

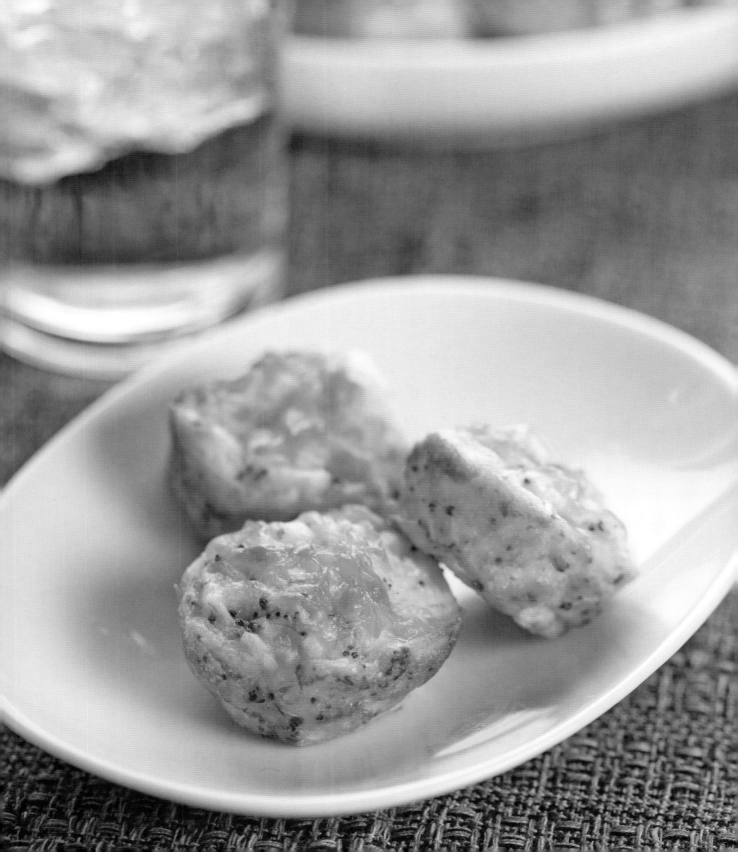

CARAMELIZED BRUSSELS SPROUTS WITH CRANBERRIES

Makes 4 servings

1 tablespoon vegetable oil

1 pound Brussels sprouts, ends trimmed and discarded, thinly sliced

¼ cup dried cranberries

2 teaspoons packed brown sugar

¼ teaspoon salt

1. Heat oil in large skillet over medium-high heat. Add Brussels sprouts; cook and stir 10 minutes or until crisp-tender and beginning to brown.

2. Add cranberries, brown sugar and salt; cook and stir 5 minutes or until Brussels sprouts are browned.

NUTRITIONAL INFORMATION

Calories **105**, Total Fat **4g**, Saturated Fat **1g**, Cholesterol **0mg**, Sodium **317mg**, Carbohydrates **17g**, Dietary Fiber **4g**, Protein **3g**

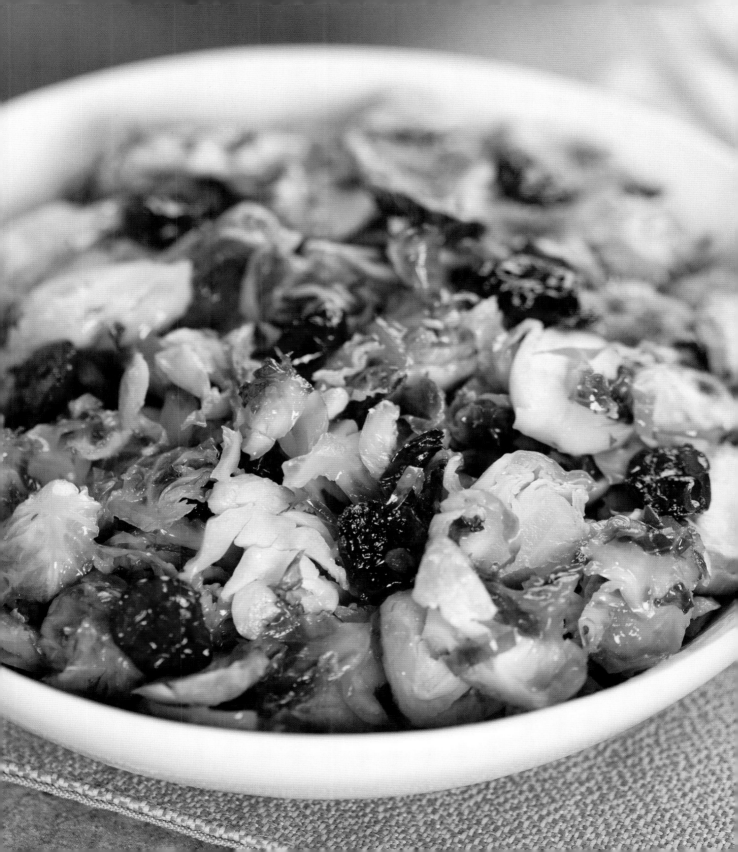

QUICK BROCCOLI SOUP

Makes 6 servings

4 cups fat-free reduced-sodium chicken or vegetable broth

2½ pounds broccoli florets

1 onion, quartered

1 cup low-fat (1%) milk

¼ teaspoon salt (optional)

¼ cup crumbled blue cheese

1. Place broth, broccoli and onion in large saucepan; bring to a boil over high heat. Reduce heat to low; cover and simmer about 20 minutes or until vegetables are tender.

2. Purée soup in blender and return to saucepan. Add milk and salt, if desired. Add water or additional broth, if needed.

3. Ladle soup into serving bowls; sprinkle with cheese.

NUTRITIONAL INFORMATION

Calories **91**, Total Fat **2g**, Saturated Fat **1g**, Cholesterol **6mg**, Sodium **175mg**, Carbohydrates **12g**, Dietary Fiber **3g**, Protein **7g**

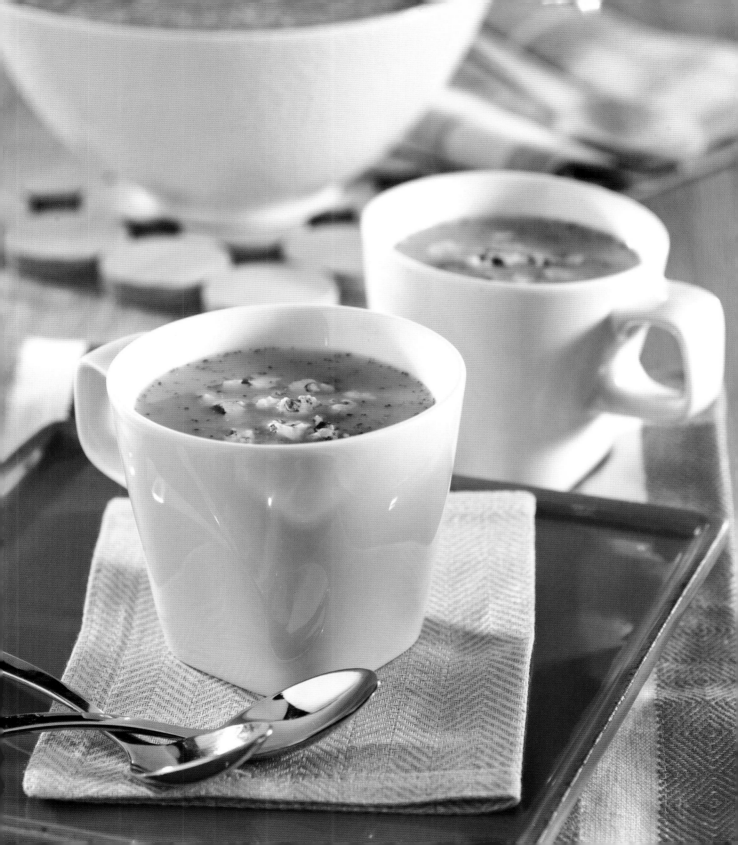

QUINOA & ROASTED VEGETABLES

Makes 6 servings

2 medium sweet potatoes, cut into ½-inch-thick slices

1 medium eggplant, peeled and cut into ½-inch cubes

1 medium tomato, cut into wedges

1 large green bell pepper, sliced

1 small onion, cut into wedges

½ teaspoon salt

¼ teaspoon black pepper

¼ teaspoon ground red pepper

1 cup uncooked quinoa

2 cloves garlic, minced

½ teaspoon dried thyme

¼ teaspoon dried marjoram

2 cups water or fat-free reduced-sodium vegetable broth

1. Preheat oven to 450°F. Line large jelly-roll pan with foil; spray with nonstick cooking spray.

2. Combine sweet potatoes, eggplant, tomato, bell pepper and onion on prepared pan; spray lightly with cooking spray. Sprinkle with salt, black pepper and ground red pepper; toss to coat. Spread vegetables in single layer. Roast 20 to 30 minutes or until vegetables are browned and tender.

3. Meanwhile, place quinoa in fine-mesh strainer; rinse well under cold running water. Spray medium saucepan with cooking spray; heat over medium heat. Add garlic, thyme and marjoram; cook and stir 1 to 2 minutes. Add quinoa; cook and stir 2 to 3 minutes. Stir in 2 cups water; bring to a boil over high heat. Reduce heat to low. Simmer, covered, 15 to 20 minutes or until water is absorbed. (Quinoa will appear somewhat translucent.) Transfer quinoa to large bowl; gently stir in roasted vegetables.

NUTRITIONAL INFORMATION

Calories **193**, Total Fat **2g**, Saturated Fat **1g**, Cholesterol **0mg**, Sodium **194mg**, Carbohydrates **40g**, Dietary Fiber **6g**, Protein **6g**

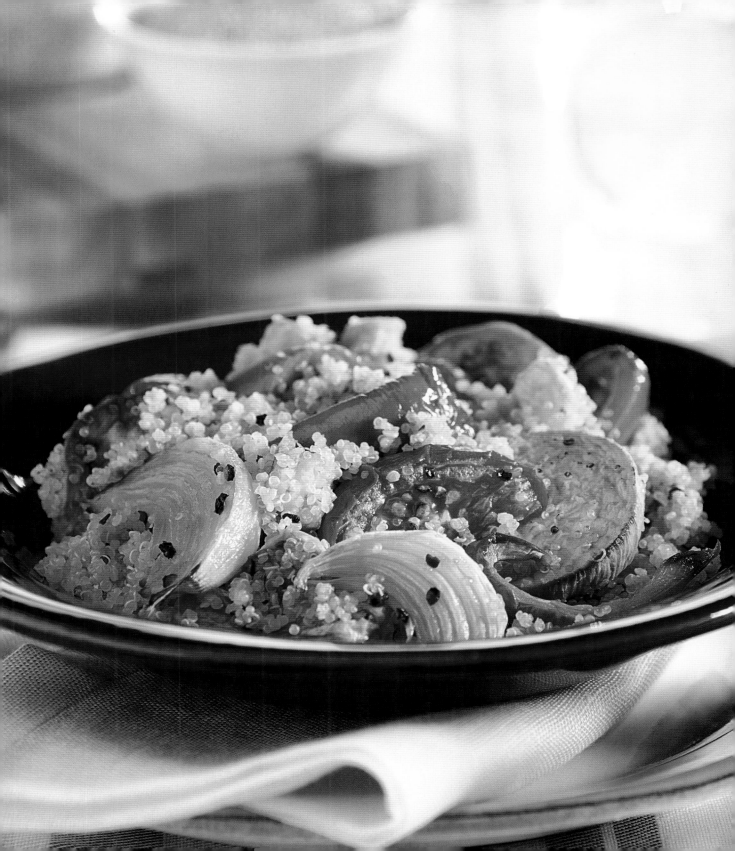

MEDITERRANEAN ORZO AND VEGETABLE PILAF

Makes 6 servings

4 ounces (½ cup plus 2 tablespoons) uncooked orzo pasta

2 teaspoons olive oil

1 small onion, diced

2 cloves garlic, minced

1 small zucchini, diced

½ cup fat-free reduced-sodium chicken broth

1 can (about 14 ounces) artichoke hearts, drained and quartered

1 medium tomato, chopped

½ teaspoon dried oregano

½ teaspoon salt

¼ teaspoon black pepper

½ cup crumbled feta cheese

Sliced black olives (optional)

1. Cook orzo according to package directions, omitting salt and fat. Drain.

2. Heat oil in large nonstick skillet over medium heat. Add onion; cook and stir 5 minutes or until translucent. Add garlic; cook and stir 1 minute. Reduce heat to low. Add zucchini and broth; simmer 5 minutes or until zucchini is crisp-tender.

3. Add cooked orzo, artichokes, tomato, oregano, salt and pepper; cook and stir 1 minute or until heated through. Top with cheese and olives, if desired.

NOTE: This makes a nice side dish to any plain grilled or roasted chicken or fish.

TIP: To reduce the sodium in this recipe, omit the salt. With all the different fresh flavors, you will not miss the extra salt.

NUTRITIONAL INFORMATION

Calories **168**, Total Fat **7g**, Saturated Fat **2g**, Cholesterol **11mg**, Sodium **516mg**, Carbohydrates **23g**, Dietary Fiber **3g**, Protein **7g**

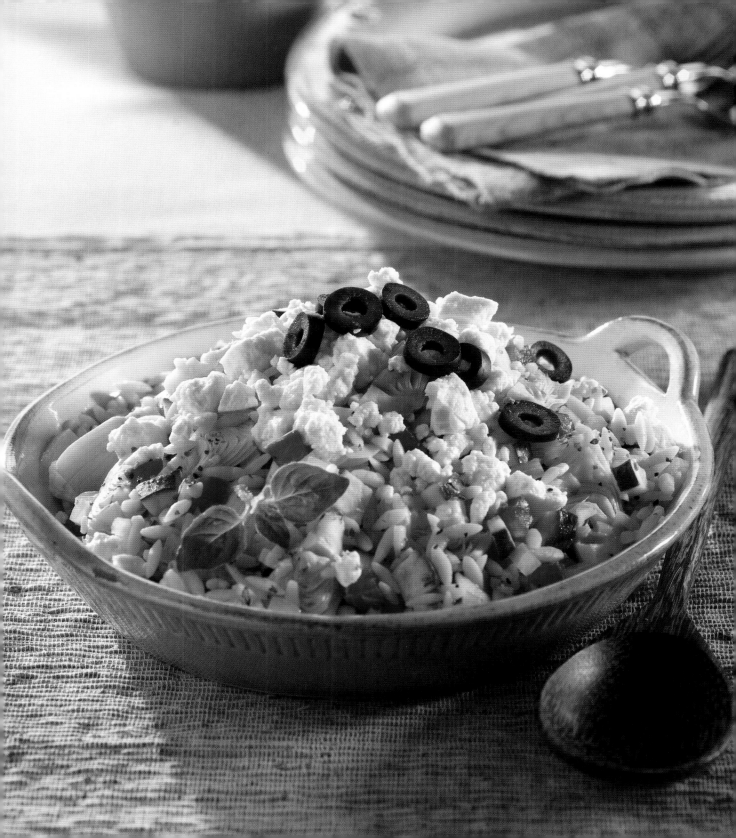

CARROT RAISIN SALAD
WITH CITRUS DRESSING

Makes 8 servings

¾ cup light sour cream

¼ cup fat-free (skim) milk

1 tablespoon honey

1 tablespoon lime juice

1 tablespoon thawed frozen
   orange juice concentrate

Grated peel of 1 medium orange

¼ teaspoon salt

8 medium carrots, peeled and
   coarsely shredded (about
   2 cups)

¼ cup raisins

⅓ cup chopped cashew nuts

1. Whisk sour cream, milk, honey, lime juice, orange juice concentrate, orange peel and salt in small bowl until smooth and well blended.

2. Combine carrots and raisins in large bowl. Add dressing; toss to coat. Cover and refrigerate 30 minutes. Gently toss before serving. Top with cashews.

NUTRITIONAL INFORMATION

Calories **127**, Total Fat **5g**, Saturated Fat **2g**, Cholesterol **8mg**, Sodium **119mg**, Carbohydrates **19g**, Dietary Fiber **3g**, Protein **4g**

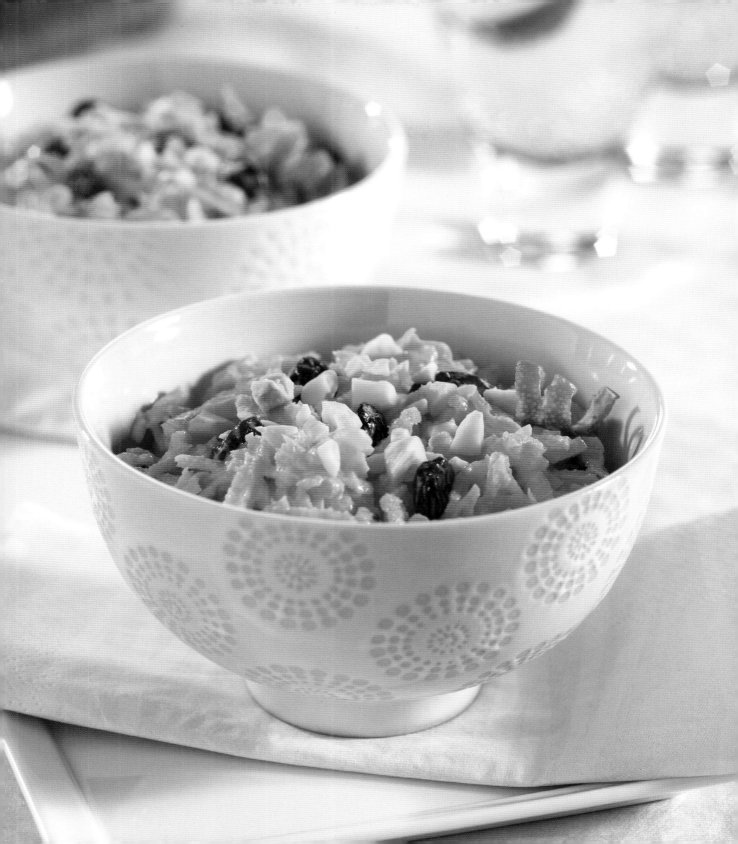

5-MINUTE HEAT-AND-GO SOUP

Makes 3½ cups (4 servings)

1 can (about 15 ounces) no-salt-added navy beans, rinsed and drained

1 can (about 14 ounces) diced tomatoes with green peppers and onions

1 cup water

1½ teaspoons dried basil

½ teaspoon sugar

½ teaspoon chicken bouillon granules

2 teaspoons olive oil

1. Place all ingredients except oil in medium saucepan; bring to a boil over high heat. Reduce heat and simmer 5 minutes, uncovered. Remove from heat; stir in oil.

2. To transport, place hot soup in vacuum flask or allow to cool and place in a plastic microwavable container. Reheat in microwave when needed.

NUTRITIONAL INFORMATION

Calories **148**, Total Fat **3g**, Saturated Fat **1g**, Cholesterol **1mg**, Sodium **451mg**, Carbohydrates **25g**, Dietary Fiber **8g**, Protein **7g**

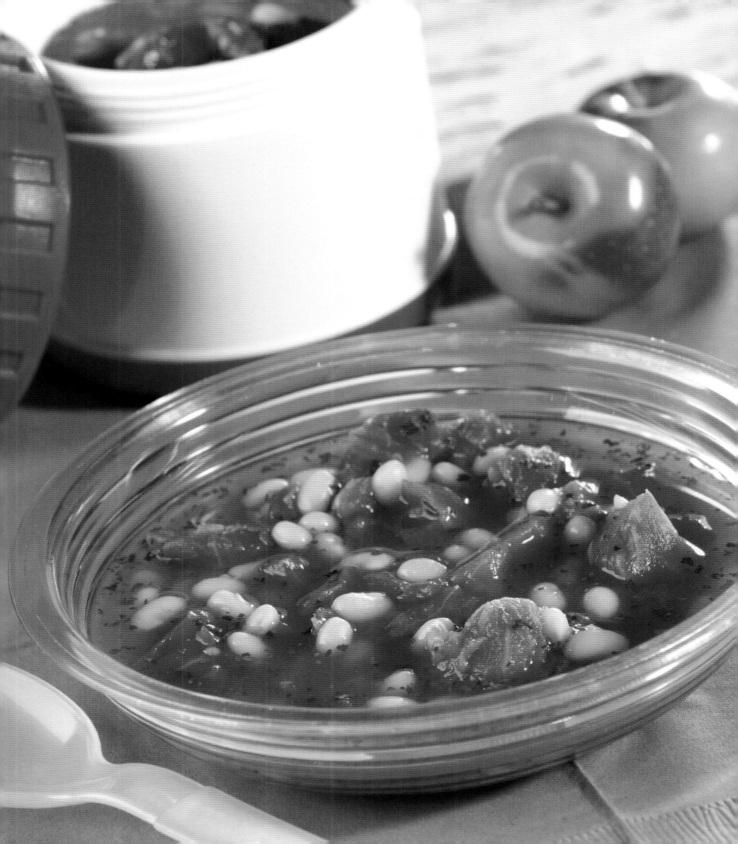

SZECHUAN EGGPLANT

Makes 4 servings

1 pound Asian eggplants or regular eggplant, peeled

2 tablespoons peanut or vegetable oil

2 cloves garlic, minced

¼ teaspoon red pepper flakes *or* ½ teaspoon hot chili oil

¼ cup vegetable broth

¼ cup hoisin sauce

3 green onions, cut into 1-inch pieces

Toasted sesame seeds* (optional)

*To toast sesame seeds, spread in small skillet. Shake skillet over medium-low heat 3 minutes or until seeds begin to pop and turn golden.

1. Cut eggplant into ½-inch slices; cut each slice into ½×½-inch strips.

2. Heat wok or large nonstick skillet over medium-high heat. Add oil; heat until hot. Add eggplant, garlic and red pepper flakes; stir-fry 7 minutes or until eggplant is very tender and browned.

3. Reduce heat to medium. Add broth, hoisin sauce and green onions to wok; cook and stir 2 minutes. Sprinkle with sesame seeds, if desired.

NUTRITIONAL INFORMATION

Calories **130**, Total Fat **8g**, Saturated Fat **1.5g**, Cholesterol **0mg**, Sodium **290mg**, Carbohydrates **14g**, Dietary Fiber **3g**, Protein **2g**

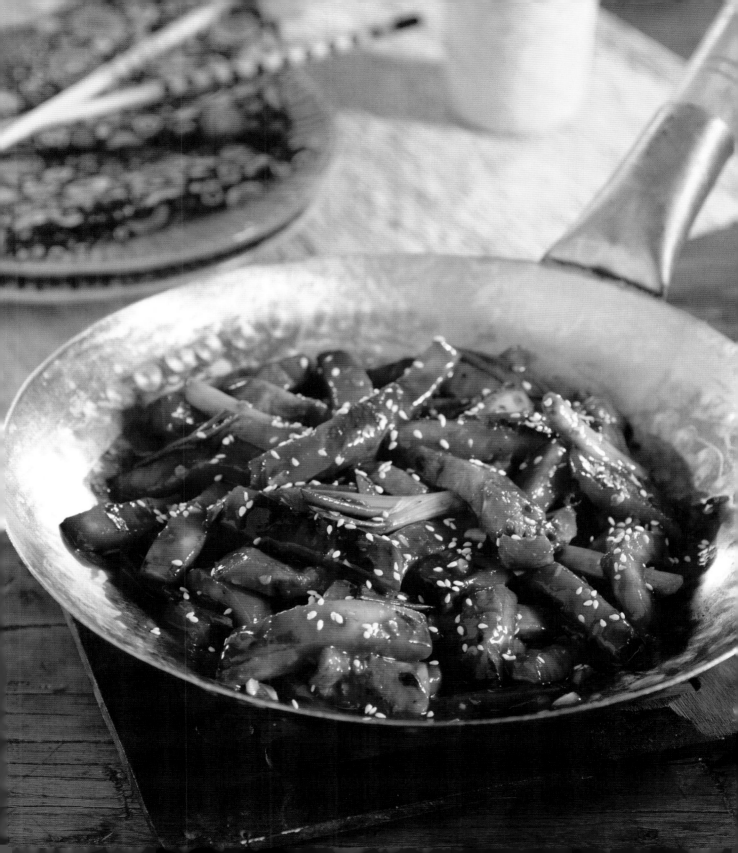

TABBOULEH IN TOMATO CUPS

Makes 8 servings

4 large firm ripe tomatoes (about 8 ounces each)

2 tablespoons olive oil

4 green onions with tops, thinly sliced diagonally, divided

1 cup uncooked bulgur wheat

1 cup water

2 tablespoons lemon juice

1 tablespoon chopped fresh mint leaves *or* ½ teaspoon dried mint

Salt and black pepper

Lemon peel and fresh mint leaves (optional)

1. Cut tomatoes in half crosswise. Scoop pulp and seeds out of tomatoes into medium bowl, leaving ¼-inch-thick shells.

2. Invert tomatoes on paper towel-lined plate; drain 20 minutes. Chop tomato pulp; set aside.

3. Heat oil in medium saucepan over medium-high heat. Cook and stir white parts of 2 onions 1 to 2 minutes until wilted. Add bulgur; cook 3 to 5 minutes until browned.

4. Add reserved tomato pulp, water, lemon juice and 1 tablespoon chopped mint to bulgur mixture. Bring to a boil over high heat; reduce heat to medium-low. Cover; simmer gently 15 to 20 minutes until liquid is absorbed.

5. Set aside a few sliced green onion tops for garnish; stir remaining 2 green onions into bulgur mixture. Season with salt and pepper. Spoon mixture into tomato cups.*

6. Preheat oven to 400°F. Place filled cups in 13×9-inch baking dish; bake 15 minutes or until heated through. Top with reserved green onion tops. Garnish with lemon peel and mint leaves. Serve immediately.

Tomato cups may be covered and refrigerated at this point up to 24 hours.

NUTRITIONAL INFORMATION

Calories **210**, Total Fat **8g**, Saturated Fat **1g**, Cholesterol **0mg**, Sodium **15mg**, Carbohydrates **34g**, Dietary Fiber **8g**, Protein **6g**

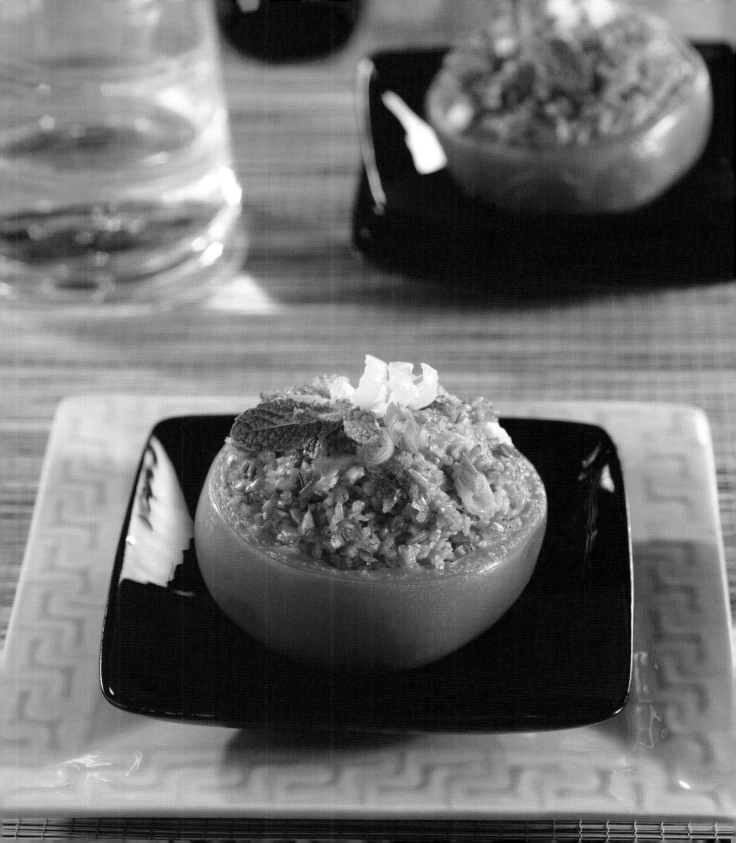

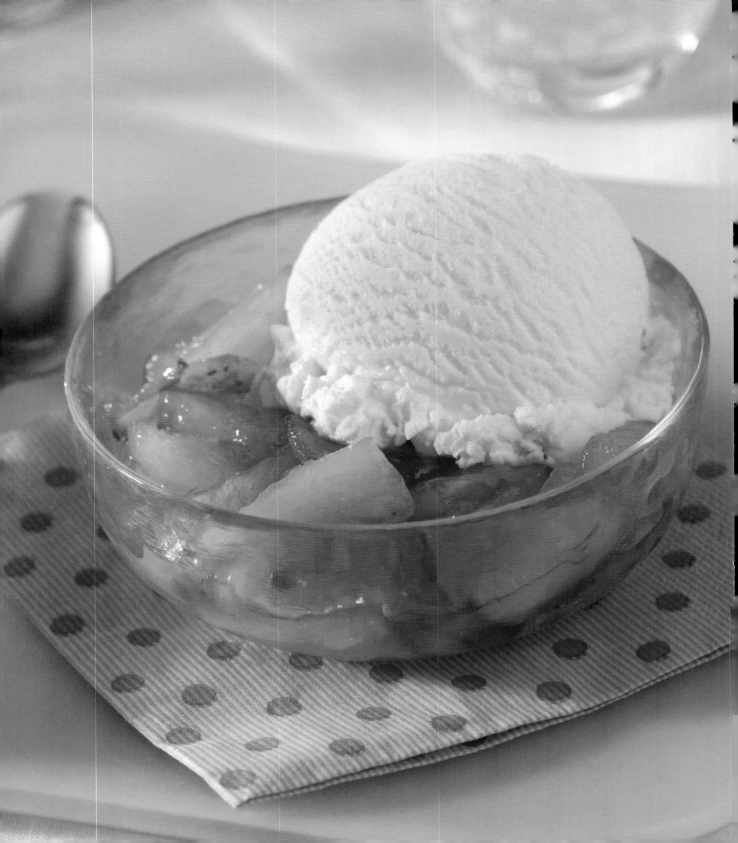

SWEETS & TREATS

CARAMELIZED PINEAPPLE

Makes 4 servings

1 tablespoon margarine

2 cups fresh pineapple chunks

3 tablespoons sugar

¾ cup vanilla reduced-fat frozen yogurt

1. Spray baking sheet with nonstick cooking spray.

2. Melt margarine in large nonstick skillet over medium-high heat. Add pineapple and sugar; cook and stir 10 to 12 minutes or until pineapple is golden brown. Spread on prepared baking sheet. Cool 5 minutes.

3. Spoon pineapple into four dessert dishes. Top each serving evenly with frozen yogurt. Serve immediately.

NUTRITIONAL INFORMATION

Calories **145**, Total Fat **4g**, Saturated Fat **1g**, Cholesterol **4mg**, Sodium **52mg**, Carbohydrates **28g**, Dietary Fiber **1g**, Protein **2g**

MUG-MADE MOCHA CAKE

Makes 1 serving

- 2 tablespoons whole wheat flour
- 2 tablespoons sugar
- 1 tablespoon cocoa powder, plus additional for garnish
- 1½ to 2 teaspoons instant coffee granules
- 1 egg white

- 3 tablespoons fat-free (skim) milk
- 1 teaspoon vegetable oil
- 2 teaspoons mini semisweet chocolate chips
- 1 tablespoon frozen fat-free whipped topping, thawed

MICROWAVE DIRECTIONS

1. Combine flour, sugar, 1 tablespoon cocoa and coffee granules in large ceramic* microwavable mug; mix well. Whisk egg white, milk and oil in small bowl until well blended. Stir into flour mixture until smooth. Fold in chocolate chips.

2. Microwave on HIGH 2 minutes. Let stand 1 to 2 minutes before serving. Top with whipped topping and additional cocoa, if desired.

This cake will only work in a ceramic mug as the material allows for more even cooking than glass.

NUTRITIONAL INFORMATION

Calories **286**, Total Fat **8g**, Saturated Fat **2g**, Cholesterol **1mg**, Sodium **80mg**, Carbohydrates **50g**, Dietary Fiber **4g**, Protein **9g**

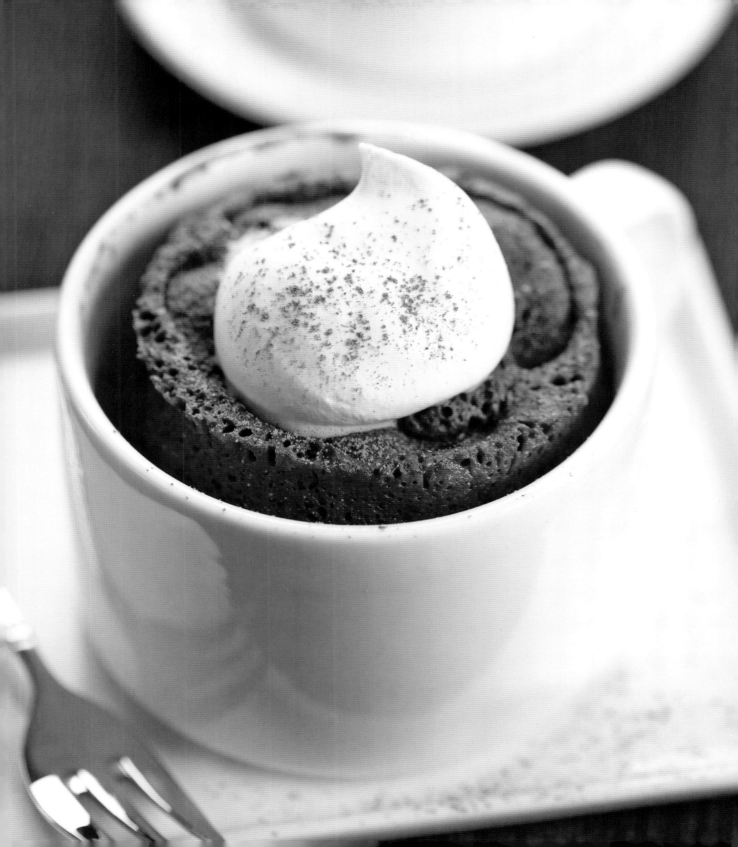

PEAR-TOPPED GRAHAMS

Makes 4 servings

¼ cup reduced-fat cream cheese

4 whole cinnamon graham crackers

4 teaspoons raspberry fruit spread

1 pear, halved, cored and cut into 16 slices

Spread 1 tablespoon cream cheese evenly over each whole cracker. Spoon 1 teaspoon fruit spread on top of each. Arrange 4 pear slices overlapping slightly on top of each cracker. Serve immediately.

NUTRITIONAL INFORMATION

Calories **127**, Total Fat **4g**, Saturated Fat **2g**, Cholesterol **10mg**, Sodium **127mg**, Carbohydrates **21g**, Dietary Fiber **2g**, Protein **3g**

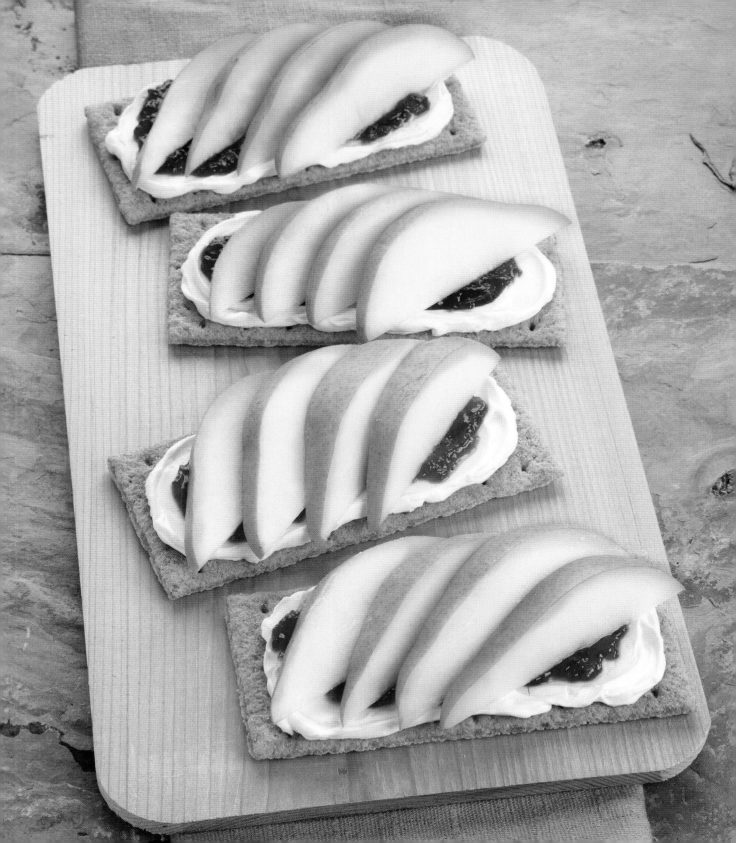

BANANA SPLIT BITES

Makes 8 servings (2 bites per serving)

1 ripe medium banana, cut into 16 slices

16 frozen mini phyllo tart shells, thawed

3 tablespoons sugar-free chocolate syrup

1 cup thawed frozen sugar-free whipped topping

1 ounce unsalted peanuts or slivered almonds, toasted* and chopped

8 maraschino cherries, halved

*To toast peanuts, spread in single layer in heavy skillet. Cook over medium heat 1 to 2 minutes or until nuts are lightly browned, stirring frequently.

Place one banana slice in each tart shell. Top with about ¾ teaspoon chocolate syrup and 1 tablespoon whipped topping. Sprinkle evenly with nuts and top with cherry half. Serve immediately or refrigerate up to 1 hour.

NUTRITIONAL INFORMATION

Calories **167**, Total Fat **7g**, Saturated Fat **3g**, Cholesterol **23mg**, Sodium **43mg**, Carbohydrates **23g**, Dietary Fiber **1g**, Protein **3g**

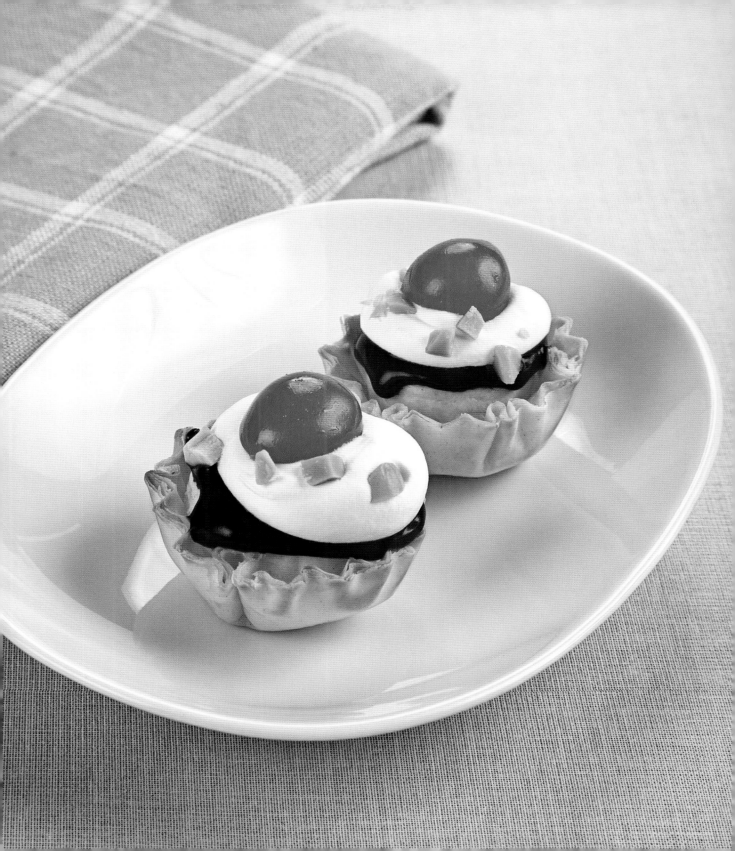

SAUTÉED APPLES SUPREME

Makes 2 servings

2 small apples *or* 1 large apple

1 teaspoon butter

¼ cup unsweetened apple juice or cider

2 teaspoons brown sugar substitute

½ teaspoon ground cinnamon

⅔ cup fat-free no-sugar-added vanilla ice cream or frozen yogurt (optional)

1 tablespoon chopped walnuts, toasted

1. Cut apples into quarters; remove cores and cut into ½-inch-thick slices.

2. Melt butter in large nonstick skillet over medium heat. Add apples; cook 4 minutes, stirring occasionally.

3. Combine apple juice, brown sugar substitute and cinnamon in small bowl; pour over apples. Simmer 5 minutes or until apples are tender and sauce thickens. Transfer to serving bowls; serve with ice cream, if desired. Sprinkle with walnuts.

NUTRITIONAL INFORMATION

Calories **139**, Total Fat **5g**, Saturated Fat **2g**, Cholesterol **6mg**, Sodium **22mg**, Carbohydrates **26g**, Dietary Fiber **4g**, Protein **1g**

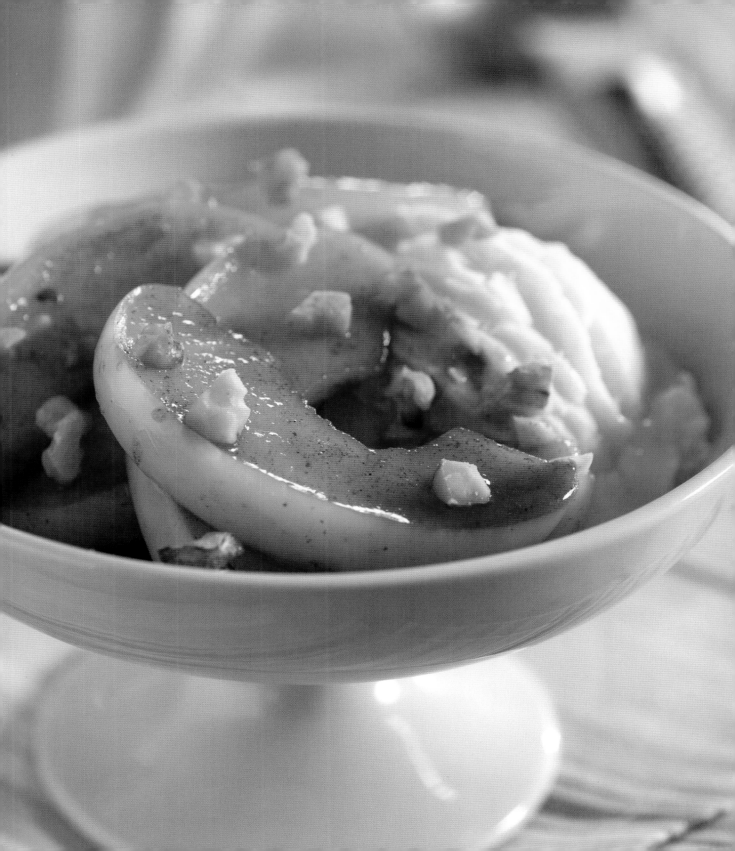

PUMPKIN SPICE MUG CAKE

Makes 1 serving

¼ cup angel food cake mix

3 tablespoons water

2 teaspoons solid-pack pumpkin

1 teaspoon finely chopped pecans

¼ teaspoon pumpkin pie spice

Whipped topping (optional)

Ground cinnamon and sugar (optional)

MICROWAVE DIRECTIONS

1. Combine cake mix, water, pumpkin, pecans and pumpkin pie spice in large ceramic* microwavable mug; mix well.

2. Microwave on HIGH 2 minutes. Let stand 1 to 2 minutes before serving. Garnish with whipped topping; sprinkle with cinnamon and sugar, if desired.

This cake will only work in a ceramic mug as the material allows for more even cooking than glass.

NUTRITIONAL INFORMATION

Calories **146**, Total Fat **2g**, Saturated Fat **0g**, Cholesterol **0mg**, Sodium **284mg**, Carbohydrates **31g**, Dietary Fiber **1g**, Protein **3g**

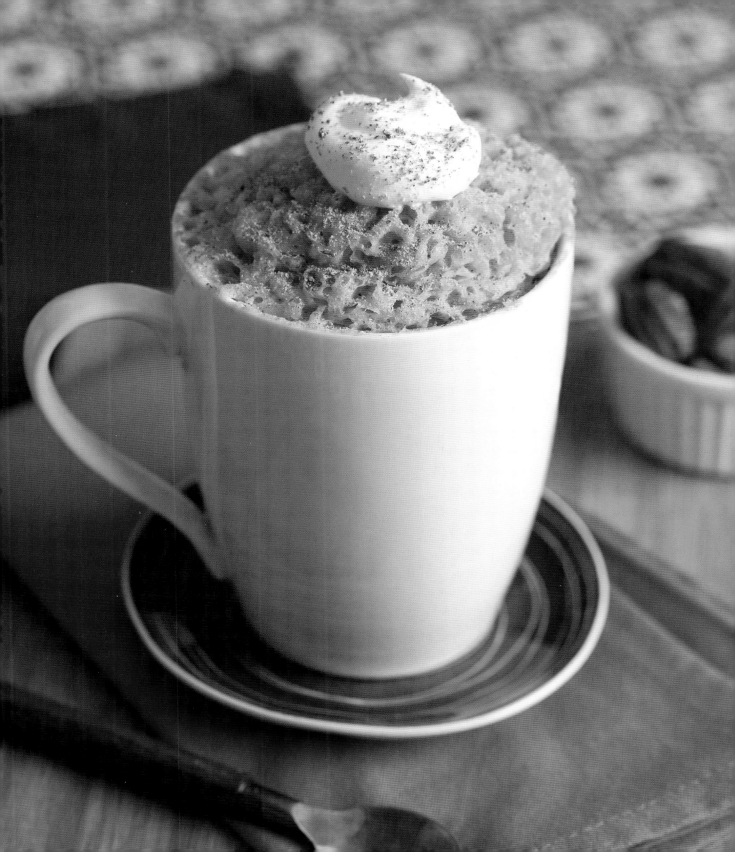

MINI ICE CREAM SANDWICHES

Makes 4 servings

8 sugar-free almond-flavored cookies

2 tablespoons all-natural strawberry fruit spread

8 strawberry slices (about 3 whole strawberries)

½ cup fat-free no-sugar-added vanilla ice cream

1. Arrange cookies, smooth side-up, on work surface. Spoon equal amounts of fruit spread on each cookie. Place 2 strawberry slices on top of 4 of the cookies.

2. Working quickly, spoon 2 tablespoons ice cream on top of strawberries, gently top with another cookie, spread side down. Place cookie sandwich on plate in freezer. Repeat with remaining ingredients. Freeze at least 30 minutes before serving.

VARIATION: Try peach or nectarine slices instead of strawberries.

NUTRITIONAL INFORMATION

Calories **254**, Total Fat **12g**, Saturated Fat **3g**, Cholesterol **3mg**, Sodium **98mg**, Carbohydrates **39g**, Dietary Fiber **1g**, Protein **3g**

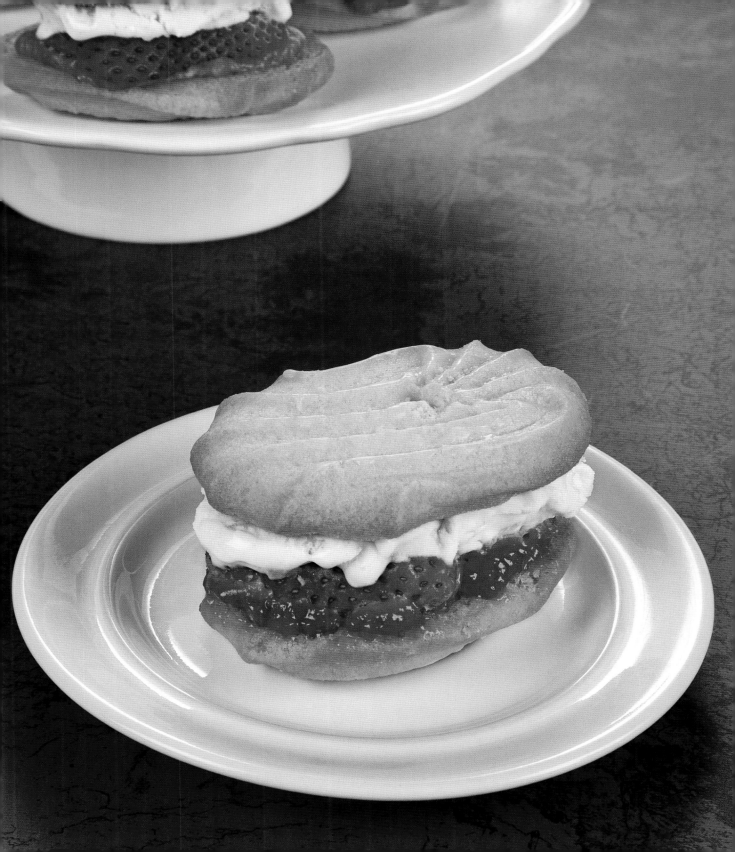

CHOCOLATE PEANUT BUTTER TRUFFLES

Makes 20 truffles (4 truffles per serving)

½ cup reduced-fat chunky peanut butter

3 tablespoons sugar substitute*

1 cup crisp rice cereal

3 tablespoons unsweetened cocoa powder

¼ cup mini semisweet chocolate chips

This recipe was tested using sucralose-based sugar substitute.

MICROWAVE DIRECTIONS

1. Place peanut butter in small microwavable bowl. Microwave on HIGH 10 seconds. Stir in sugar substitute with wooden spoon until smooth. Stir in cereal; mix well.

2. Line large plate with waxed paper. Spray hands with nonstick cooking spray; shape peanut butter mixture into 1-inch balls, pressing firmly. Place balls on prepared plate; freeze 15 minutes or up to 1 hour.

3. Spread cocoa on small plate. Roll each truffle in cocoa; return to large plate.

4. Place chocolate chips in small resealable food storage bag. Microwave on HIGH 10 seconds; knead bag. Repeat until chocolate is melted and smooth.

5. Press melted chocolate into one corner of bag; cut very small hole in corner. Drizzle chocolate over truffles. Let chocolate set before serving. Truffles can be refrigerated in airtight container up to 3 days.

NUTRITIONAL INFORMATION

Calories **220**, Total Fat **12g**, Saturated Fat **3g**, Cholesterol **0mg**, Sodium **229mg**, Carbohydrates **25g**, Dietary Fiber **3g**, Protein **8g**

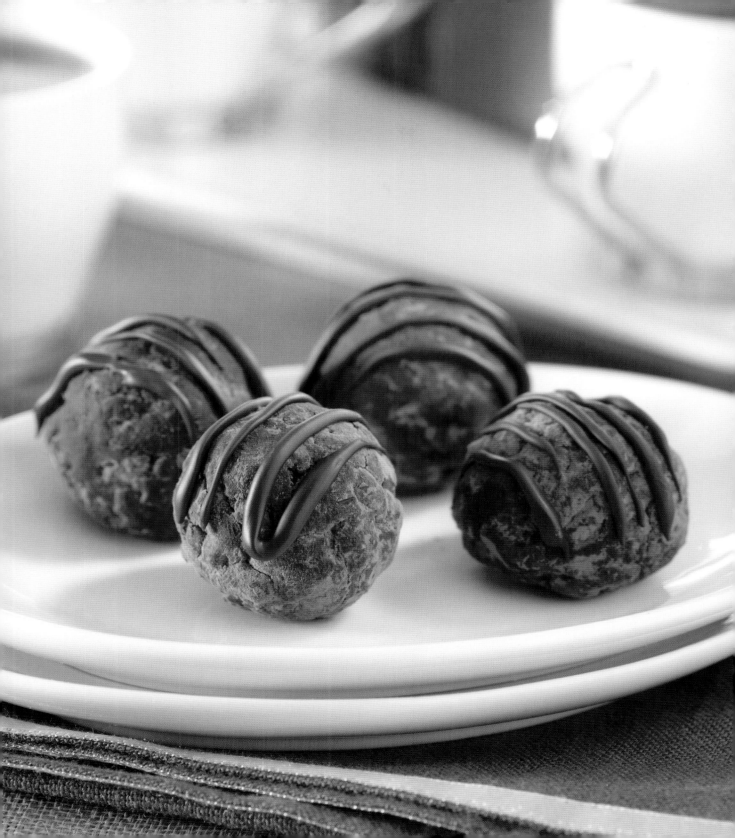

POACHED PEARS IN CINNAMON-APRICOT SAUCE

Makes 4 servings

1 can (5½ ounces) apricot nectar

1 tablespoon sugar

1 teaspoon lemon juice

½ teaspoon ground cinnamon

¼ teaspoon grated lemon peel

⅛ teaspoon ground cloves

2 large pears

Fat-free whipped topping (optional)

1. Combine apricot nectar, sugar, lemon juice, cinnamon, lemon peel and cloves in large skillet. Bring to a boil over medium-high heat.

2. Meanwhile, cut pears lengthwise into halves, leaving stem attached to one half. Remove cores. Cut pears lengthwise into thin slices, taking care not to cut through stem end. Add pears to skillet with nectar mixture; return to a boil. Reduce heat to medium-low. Simmer, covered, 6 to 8 minutes or just until pears are tender. Carefully remove pears from skillet, reserving liquid.

3. Simmer liquid in skillet, uncovered, over medium heat 2 to 3 minutes or until mixture thickens slightly, stirring occasionally. Fan out pears; spoon sauce over pears. Serve pears warm or chilled with whipped topping, if desired.

NUTRITIONAL INFORMATION

Calories **84**, Total Fat **1g**, Saturated Fat **1g**, Cholesterol **0mg**, Sodium **1mg**, Carbohydrates **22g**, Dietary Fiber **3g**, Protein **1g**

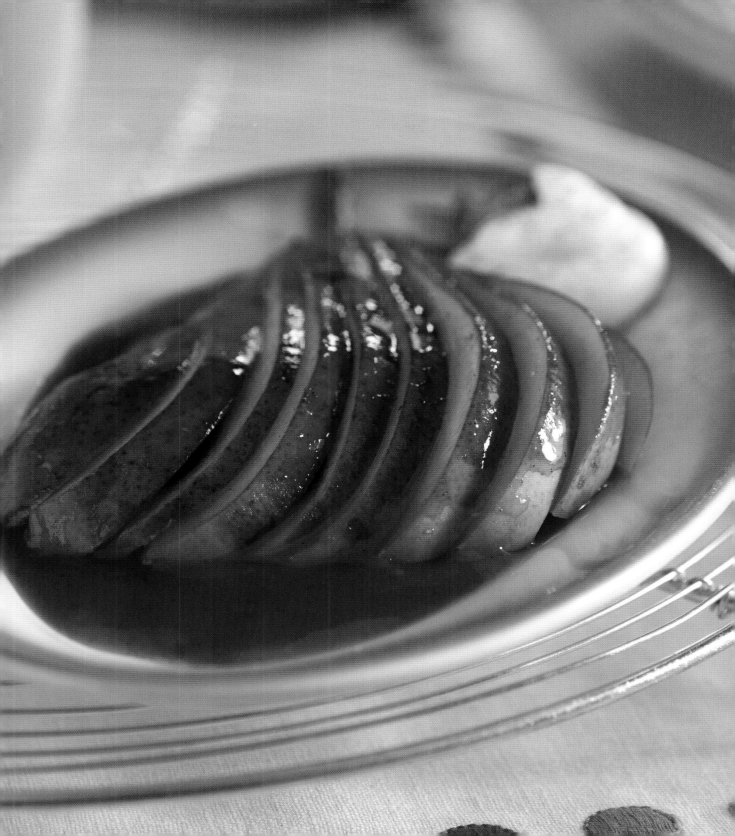

VANILLA PUMPKIN PIE

Makes 8 servings

1 package (4-serving size) fat-free, sugar-free vanilla instant pudding and pie filling mix

1½ cups fat-free (skim) milk

1 cup canned pumpkin

1 teaspoon sugar substitute

¼ teaspoon ground cinnamon

¼ teaspoon ground nutmeg

1 baked 8-inch reduced-fat pie crust

1. Whisk pudding mix and milk in medium bowl until well blended. Add pumpkin, sugar substitute, cinnamon and nutmeg; mix well.

2. Pour filling into crust. Refrigerate 3 hours or until firm.

TIP: Make this recipe the day before and refrigerate overnight.

NUTRITIONAL INFORMATION

Calories **158**, Total Fat **8g**, Saturated Fat **2g**, Cholesterol **1mg**, Sodium **308mg**, Carbohydrates **19g**, Dietary Fiber **1g**, Protein **3g**

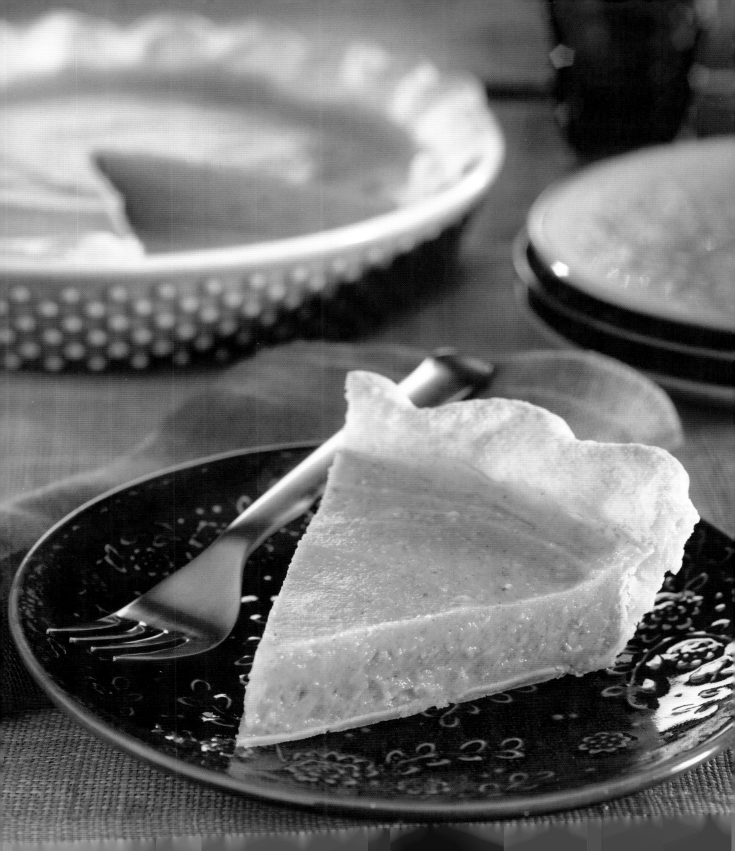

STRAWBERRY CHEESECAKE PARFAITS

Makes 4 servings

1½ cups vanilla nonfat Greek yogurt

½ cup whipped cream cheese, at room temperature

2 tablespoons powdered sugar

1 teaspoon vanilla

2 cups sliced fresh strawberries

2 teaspoons granulated sugar

8 honey graham cracker squares, coarsely crumbled (about 2 cups)

Fresh mint leaves (optional)

1. Whisk yogurt, cream cheese, powdered sugar and vanilla in small bowl until smooth and well blended.

2. Combine strawberries and granulated sugar in small bowl; gently toss.

3. Layer ¼ cup yogurt mixture, ¼ cup strawberries and ¼ cup graham cracker crumbs in each of four dessert dishes. Repeat layers. Garnish with mint. Serve immediately.

NUTRITIONAL INFORMATION

Calories **220**, Total Fat **7g**, Saturated Fat **3g**, Cholesterol **15mg**, Sodium **200mg**, Carbohydrates **29g**, Dietary Fiber **2g**, Protein **11g**

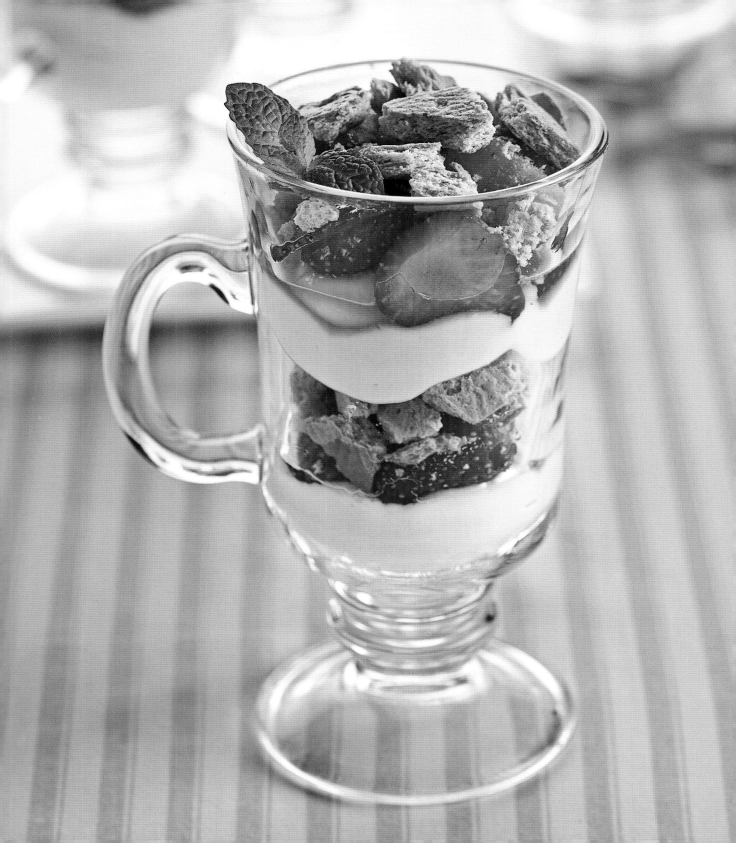

FRUIT SALAD with CREAMY BANANA DRESSING

Makes 8 servings

2 cups fresh pineapple chunks

1 cup cantaloupe cubes

1 cup honeydew melon cubes

1 cup fresh blackberries

1 cup sliced fresh strawberries

1 cup seedless red grapes

1 medium apple, diced

2 medium ripe bananas, sliced

½ cup vanilla nonfat Greek yogurt

2 tablespoons honey

1 tablespoon fresh lemon juice

¼ teaspoon ground nutmeg

1. Combine pineapple, cantaloupe, honeydew, blackberries, strawberries, grapes and apple in large bowl; mix gently.

2. Combine bananas, yogurt, honey, lemon juice and nutmeg in blender or food processor; blend until smooth.

3. Pour dressing over fruit mixture; gently toss to coat. Serve immediately.

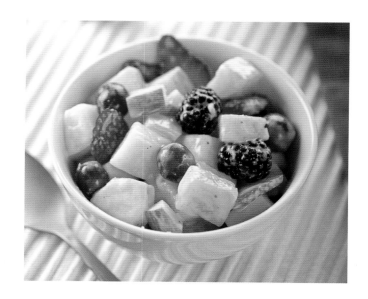

NUTRITIONAL INFORMATION

Calories **125**, Total Fat **0g**, Saturated Fat **0g**, Cholesterol **0mg**, Sodium **15mg**, Carbohydrates **31g**, Dietary Fiber **4g**, Protein **3g**

INDEX

• INDEX •

• INDEX •

• METRIC CONVERSION CHART •

VOLUME MEASUREMENTS (dry)

1/8 teaspoon = 0.5 mL
1/4 teaspoon = 1 mL
1/2 teaspoon = 2 mL
3/4 teaspoon = 4 mL
1 teaspoon = 5 mL
1 tablespoon = 15 mL
2 tablespoons = 30 mL
1/4 cup = 60 mL
1/3 cup = 75 mL
1/2 cup = 125 mL
2/3 cup = 150 mL
3/4 cup = 175 mL
1 cup = 250 mL
2 cups = 1 pint = 500 mL
3 cups = 750 mL
4 cups = 1 quart = 1 L

VOLUME MEASUREMENTS (fluid)

1 fluid ounce (2 tablespoons) = 30 mL
4 fluid ounces (1/2 cup) = 125 mL
8 fluid ounces (1 cup) = 250 mL
12 fluid ounces (1 1/2 cups) = 375 mL
16 fluid ounces (2 cups) = 500 mL

WEIGHTS (mass)

1/2 ounce = 15 g
1 ounce = 30 g
3 ounces = 90 g
4 ounces = 120 g
8 ounces = 225 g
10 ounces = 285 g
12 ounces = 360 g
16 ounces = 1 pound = 450 g

DIMENSIONS

1/16 inch = 2 mm
1/8 inch = 3 mm
1/4 inch = 6 mm
1/2 inch = 1.5 cm
3/4 inch = 2 cm
1 inch = 2.5 cm

OVEN TEMPERATURES

250°F = 120°C
275°F = 140°C
300°F = 150°C
325°F = 160°C
350°F = 180°C
375°F = 190°C
400°F = 200°C
425°F = 220°C
450°F = 230°C

BAKING PAN SIZES

Utensil	Size in Inches/Quarts	Metric Volume	Size in Centimeters
Baking or Cake Pan (square or rectangular)	8×8×2	2 L	20×20×5
	9×9×2	2.5 L	23×23×5
	12×8×2	3 L	30×20×5
	13×9×2	3.5 L	33×23×5
Loaf Pan	8×4×3	1.5 L	20×10×7
	9×5×3	2 L	23×13×7
Round Layer Cake Pan	8×1½	1.2 L	20×4
	9×1½	1.5 L	23×4
Pie Plate	8×1¼	750 mL	20×3
	9×1¼	1 L	23×3
Baking Dish or Casserole	1 quart	1 L	—
	1½ quart	1.5 L	—
	2 quart	2 L	—